The Ultimate
Cellulite Treatment in
a Book

The Ultimate Cellulite Treatment in a Book

Bronwyn M. Hewitt

iUniverse, Inc.
New York Lincoln Shanghai

The Ultimate Cellulite Treatment in a Book

iUniverse books may be ordered through booksellers or by contacting:

iUniverse
2021 Pine Lake Road, Suite 100
Lincoln, NE 68512
www.iuniverse.com
1-800-Authors (1-800-288-4677)

Because of the dynamic nature of the Internet, any Web addresses or links contained in this book may have changed since publication and may no longer be valid.

The information, ideas, and suggestions in this book are not intended as a substitute for professional medical advice. Before following any suggestions contained in this book, you should consult your personal physician. Neither the author nor the publisher shall be liable or responsible for any loss or damage allegedly arising as a consequence of your use or application of any information or suggestions in this book.

ISBN: 978-0-595-46586-6 (pbk)
ISBN: 978-0-595-90882-0 (ebk)

Printed in the United States of America

- Michelle, my brilliant photographer, enthusiastic editor, and long-time best friend. I thank you for always supporting me in my dream to help other women. You have been there from the beginning when I was first treating people 15 years ago and you have constantly and unwaveringly believed in me. This in itself has been one of the greatest gifts of my life. [Karen, actually we know you really did the 1st edition. Thank you for saving me from the shame of my typos. I am forever in your debt.]

- My Mother Doreen, for giving me a healthy and stable start in life. And for filling my head with ol' wives tales.

- And to someone incredibly special and generous who brightened up my childhood and whom I overheard as a little girl stating "all I eat a day is one dry cracker and I still put on weight" these words have stayed with me all my life–little did I know at the time that they would encourage me towards writing this book and is the basis for my life's work to help women break free of the vicious cycle of weight gain from dieting. To my Godmother Aunty Margy Adams–thank you with all my heart for being in my life.

- And of course a special big thanks to my wonderful, patient and tireless Webmaster–Ken Dunway. www.dunway.com Without you my website would be far less than successful on account of the fact that no-one would have found it!

"Do not wait; the time will never be 'just right'.
Start where you stand, and work with whatever tools you may have at your command."

—Napoleon Hill

Contents

Important Questions For You To Consider Now

Here are some questions that I would like you to answer to get you thinking about your body and how your lifestyle choices affect your health. Maybe pencil in your answers.

Answer these questions right now, don't think about it just do it before you read on.

It will be great for you to come back again in a few months and see how your responses have changed.

Basics About You

Select a Personality that you believe describe how you are most of the time on the inside:
Happy; Vibrant; Sad; Shy; Depressed; Lively; Serious; Spontaneous.

When do you exercise?
Regularly; Never; Sometimes; Rarely;

Do you exercise?
Alone; with friends, in public; at the gym.

About Your Cellulite

How long do you think you have had cellulite?

How did you first notice you had cellulite?

Where did your cellulite first appear?

Have you tried other cellulite treatments previous to TUCT?

If so was there any improvement in your cellulite?

How long did it take for your cellulite to come back?

Your Chemical Intake

Are you aware that your body does not know what to do or how to process chemicals?

Do you eat processed foods? If so please list them.
What type of chemical products do you clean with?

What chemical products do you use on your body for personal hygiene? I.e. shower gel; deodorant.

What type of chemical products do you use on your body?
I.e. Body lotions, makeup.

Your Stress Levels

Does your job cause you undue stress? Does it follow you home?

Does your partner or their job cause you to stress or worry?

Do any members of your family raise your stress levels unnecessarily?

Are you aware that you can choose not to stress?

What tools do you use to deal with your stress levels?

If you don't have any tools yet, seek advice, ask your friends what they do, try different things until you find something that not only relieves stress but brings you joy. (This could for instance be a combination of walking and chocolate but it usually involves finding a bit of time for yourself—even 10 minutes of quiet can help).

But **beware the TREAT syndrome**. Many of us as children received treats for good behaviour from our parents and elders. This leads to you the adult giving yourself treats to make you feel better. We give ourselves treats to get that rewarding feeling that we received as a child to feel better about ourselves. So if we feel bad or stressed we cheer ourselves up with a treat. Try not to do this to your children. Instead reward them with praise. privilege or responsibility.

Three steps to relieving situational stress.

1. Change the situation

This may involve opening a line of communication with a particular person.

2. Change your attitude towards the situation or person.

This may involve honest self assessment.

3. Accept then Remove yourself from the situation, then let it go.

YOUR FEELINGS

How do you feel about your world? Safe; Fearful; Loving; Confidant; Angry.

> If you feel angry often, ask yourself what you are afraid of or what you fear may happen.

How do you feel about yourself? Safe; Fearful; Loving; Confidant; Angry.

Are your expectations of yourself high or low?

How do you feel about yourself during the week?

How do you feel about yourself on the weekend?

> If your feelings are different ask yourself why, what is fundamentally different. It could be as simple as your job or it could be and issue of control or safety.

How would you like to feel about yourself every day?

Are you aware that you can be stressed because your body physically isn't working properly?

Do you believe that if your body is physically less stressed you will be mentally less stressed as well?

Your Problems ONE AT A TIME

What is your biggest problem at this moment?

How do you feel when you think about this problem?

How would you feel if this problem went away?

If the problem went away would it change your daily life in any way?

ABOUT THE ULTIMATE CELLULITE TREATMENT

Hi, my name is Bronwyn and my background is in natural therapies, massage (Diploma Swedish Massage), back to basics food intake (Certificate of Nutrition) and the use of essential oils; and among other things; experience from treating women of all ages and all shapes and sizes.

I have been helping women in Australia lose their cellulite for over 18 years. I have operated the cellulite treatment as a hobby alongside my career in Real Estate and later in the mining industry. I have treated around 1000 women and all of them have learnt how to get rid of their cellulite successfully, all of them have at the very least experienced a major improvement in the way they look and feel. Their cellulite has been reduced and in many cases gone all together but that is up to the client, some are just happy for it to be reduced to the point of being able to wear a bikini.

My aim has always been not to keep a client forever but to teach them what I know so that they can keep their cellulite at bay on their own using the tools that I give them.

I am, I should admit as early on as possible; can be a little lazy, I would much prefer to read a book than go for a run any day, am not terribly driven and tend to aim for the easiest (and hopefully the smartest) solution to any problem I come across.

This treatment is therefore really easy.

If you've tried any of the other multitudes of cellulite treatments before reading this book, you are possibly either exhausted, confused or don't believe it is possible to eliminate your cellulite.

But you didn't give up hope. Well done. This shows me that you are in touch with your inner self, who knew that having cellulite was wrong and you can get rid of it.

I can tell you now that **it *is* possible to loose your cellulite** and very simple and easy to do.

I have had clients that have been to every known treatment on the market; (liposuction inclusive) and I will never say that they don't work but I will say that most often the reason for you having cellulite is completely overlooked and this is a major problem.

It is **vitally important** that you know what your weakness is or what part of your anatomy needs the most attention—**the cause of your cellulite**. And there are several.

Where there is an effect there is always a cause. This is the number one reason why my treatment is so effective.

With this book and my on line help at askbron@gmail.com we will find the cause of your cellulite.

The Ultimate Cellulite Treatment covers all symptoms. So no matter how you got your cellulite, you can get rid of your cellulite forever.

EVERY ONE of you has cellulite for a particular main reason. What you need to do is establish your particular reason and then deflect the cause and you're done.

Sound easy? Well it is just that. And we'll talk about how soon.

Some of the more common reasons for getting cellulite are, slow metabolism; poor circulation, digestive problems and constipation, or you are just eating foods that our bodies weren't intended to consume. These problems are interfering with your body's natural processes almost closing it down.

Find your particular weakness and you're half way there.

More about what you can do is in the chapter headed "REA-
SONS FOR STORING CELLULITE OR ENERGY".

I am going to show you how to kick start your body again so it
works at it's intended ultimate levels of performance mainly
for digestion, circulation and elimination. And it's not all hard
work, you will have fun, you will feel better, your body will be
happy.

You'll find this is not a serious book
but the results are!

My system for getting rid of your cellulite forever, is packed
full of common sense, that we all already know but have forgotten.

You will experience a lot of A-HA's (or OMIGOD's) like a
light bulb being switched on whilst reading this book, much
of what I tell you, you may feel that you already know,
because we already know the truth and I believe we (you and
I) have the world's knowledge within reach.

So when you hear the truth you may think–"hey that sounds
so right or familiar, I think I already knew that" but that
knowledge wasn't in your conscious mind and you weren't
necessarily using the information now in your every day life.

This is why the Ultimate Cellulite Treatment is so ridiculously
easy.

All you have to do is prompt your internal systems how to function as they should be doing automatically. Due to <u>environment</u>, <u>stress</u>, <u>time limitations</u> et cetera; we have put our body's on a borrowed 'fast food lifestyle' and your system is unable to function like this for long. Then problems/illnesses begin to take hold.

WHAT IS THIS CELLULITE ANYWAY?

Cellulite It is a (very) sticky glob of waste that clings to fat cells.

Waste being toxins. Toxins being from preservatives, additives, slow moving food and general chemical products that we eat or breathe or wash into our systems

The word cellulite well … it's French you know … pronounced 'sell you leet'.

Interestingly, there are a variety of meanings of cellulite as it is still a fairly new affliction as far as the medical fraternity goes.

Unfortunately it is seen as a weight problem associated with weight gain or low fitness levels when actually it is a 'diss-ease' (as opposed to disease) of your internal body and an outside sign that things are not working properly on the inside.

Men don't get cellulite because they don't have the protective hormone oestrogen that carries waste to the outer parts of the body away from the reproductive system.

Therefore it is very important for you all to note that if you have cellulite your husband may have furred up arteries.

As men don't have the protective hormone to move the toxins and waste away from their vital organs it will begin to clog up and eventually harden their arteries leading to serious health problems concerning the heart.

Hence historically men have always been more prone to heart attack–this is why. This will also affect their circulation and elimination systems.

Yep, first the beer gut, then the man boobs.

OK, so back to 'what is cellulite?'

Most people will tell you that cellulite is fat or are fat cells–if this were true, why can overweight people not have cellulite and skinny people do!

I've had many, many clients that are as thin as thin because they have tried to starve away their cellulite or pump it off in the gym, thinking it was some type of fat, but this simply can't be done.

Cellulite I believe to be waste, and by waste I mean the toxic kind.

Our bodies are not particularly good at knowing how to eliminate and then expel <u>chemicals</u>, <u>additives</u>, <u>preservatives</u> and other unnatural products.

We simply weren't designed when these things existed.

We may in time evolve into an organism that is able to handle such unnatural products, but this won't happen in my lifetime, your children's or your great, great grandchildren's!

And because we find it difficult to eliminate toxins, impurities, unnatural foods and additives, our body's protective system sends them to the outer parts of the body where they cling on to the fat cell and if you think about it this is the safest place for them to be where they can cause no harm to the vital organs and systems in the rest of the body.

These days communities are recycling more and more but there is still so much that we just leave at the tip as some rubbish can't be recycled and so just gets dumped at the tip. Imagine that your thighs are this tip; full of stuff we are unable to recycle.

It is time to empty your body's rubbish tip.

In saying this, you could quite understandably figure; 'well if I just cover up and no one can see my cellulite it is not detrimental to my health, as it is being kept in a relatively safe place—this problem is only cosmetic'.

But as with all signs that the body shows us indicating that something is wrong internally, cellulite is another such warning sign. Luckily we can see our cellulite, and it is an indication that we are clogging up our systems and are therefore not eliminating waste properly.

This causes a vicious cycle, and as the body becomes more and more sluggish in all its systems, eliminatory, digestive, circulatory, et cetera, the body slows down and works less than well. Then bad things start to happen to us.
We get sick more often, we catch colds and allergies more easily, we put on weight and we lose our energy levels at an alarming rate AND as the brain is just another organ, we may cope less well in our day to day lives, reacting unreasonably to stress and change, and in some cases we can become despondent and even depressed.

In many cases where I have treated a lady for her cellulite, the treatment becomes a holistic treatment, as every part of you—physical, mental, and spiritual—begins to shine, and one member of the family treating their cellulite can heal an entire family.

As we all know when Mum is happy the whole family is happy. *Right girls?!*

If you are not overweight and are wondering what your cellulite is clinging to, I'll explain.

Everyone has a specific number of fat cells.

An overweight person does not have more fat cells than a skinny person. They simply have larger ones.
So for those of the lean variety who have cellulite, it is also hanging on to your fat cells. So **everyone has fat cells—if you loose weight you don't loose cells, they simply get smaller**.

Cellulite and stored energy are like a layer of gooey stuff under the skin. When you have a lot, it can be quite solid and those bumps and lumps may not be too obvious.

So when you start to loose the cellulite from your stored energy, those lumps and bumps may tend to appear worse as they break down and separate, and as they become fewer they can also become more pronounced.

Now DON"T PANIC, although in saying this, many of you will still email me with the proverbial "Aaaaaaaaaaagggggghh-hhh my cellulite is looking worse!!!!"

I understand your fears but truly, **this is a great sign that the cellulite is loosening, moving, and becoming less and less present**, and those more stubborn lumps that are taking a bit longer seem to stick out more, so give those a good twiddling.

This stage is actually one worth noting and celebrating, as it means that all your systems are working and you can be happy and very proud of yourself.

If you are doing this treatment during the warmer months, invest in a couple of gorgeous sarongs and cotton ¾-length pants. Please try to avoid shorts at all costs; very few (0.00001%) people look good in shorts. If you do, go for a longer-leg cargo design. The details and small pockets everywhere are very slimming.

A BIT OF MY HISTORY

Back in the good old days when I was about 24 years old–oh don't get me wrong, at 41 the days are still good days, too, but you know what I mean …

Anyway, around this time I did an early sea change. I moved out of the city and into the hills. I had been living in the fast lane and wanted out.

I had ugly, wobbly and bumpy thighs and I wasn't happy. As someone who always had an interest in health and massage, and had studied both subjects, I decided to look into this problem of cellulite.

I researched and read articles on cellulite and investigated the treatments available. No one seemed to be able to tell me what it is, and even worse, no one was able to get rid of it!

Some of the treatments out there were and still are almost bar-baric! People were suffering much bruising to their legs and their egos, l was often told by ladies that when a treatment was not working clients were generally told it was their own fault; that they must be doing something wrong–just awful.

So I moved away from modern technology, as I wasn't getting any answers there, or at least certainly not the answers I wanted, they just didn't feel right.

I turned to the world of natural therapies and much to my delight I found slowly and surely, piece by piece, the answers I had been looking for.

My research and processing of information lasted for over two years, and what I learned over that time made so much sense, and still make up the foundations of what you are about to learn.

When I first began treating women in the late 80s, I soon discovered that not only did my treatment work, but it was actually quite quick, and affected people in ways I had not foreseen.

Women stopped getting <u>headaches</u>, <u>period pain</u>, their <u>stress disappeared</u>.

Women were generally happier and functioned better, and in many cases this affected their entire family.

Helping women help themselves is now my life's work.

As my treatment developed over the years, so too, did the name. The first name was The Smooth Move. There was another company also called The Smooth Move at the time, which was a furniture removal company, and my friends and family took great delight in reminding me of this.

Later the treatment became The Hewitt Home Cellulite Treatment—yep pretty original, hey? My favourite came later, which was Naturally Better. I am still fond of that one but when it came time to name the book and the website for global distribution I wanted the name to say more.

I knew that I had developed the ultimate treatment for cellulite simply because it was so effective, it worked, and the cellulite stayed away.

The Ultimate Cellulite Treatment is just that
Ultimate.

To be sure I looked up the word ultimate and according to Roget's Thesaurus *ultimate* represents:

Final	if this treatment is your last resort, then good for you—this is the last and final treatment you will ever need.
Eventual	is now—you will cleanse away your cellulite for ever
Decisive	this will be the easiest decision you've ever made
Definitive	this treatment is tried and tested

Vital	not only will your legs look great, this treatment is vital for you and your family's health.
Crucial	if you have cellulite the alpha males in your family will more than likely have hardened or furred up arteries.

So he and **the whole family will benefit** |
Critical	your health is in a risky state.
First	if you're lucky this will be your first; last and ONLY treatment
Fundamental	best you don't break that word down into syllables! But this is a very back to basics natural treatment to get rid of your cellulite and is therefore ridiculously easy
Basic	back to basics is where you and I will go together
Essential	the oils you will use are just essential, not fragrant
Supreme	yes you can still eat Pizza
Extreme	extremely better than you've ever felt is just around your corner
Greatest	at the end of this treatment you may just consider yourself to be the greatest person you know
Best	you will be 'the bestest' you can be. It's so easy.

Really it is.

What you will read in this book is the knowledge I have gained from the experience of researching, developing and treating women with cellulite. I have many theories and beliefs and they are just that. But this is what is known to me and what works.

I am delighted and thrilled about this opportunity to share it with you and I can also say that this treatment has worked for EVERYBODY.

I don't like to say it is 100% successful as it is too hard for people to believe but I can tell you that I am yet to meet someone that the treatment has had no effect on.

It is natural, gentle and it does work.

So here you are at the end of my intro. In the next few chapters I will give you everything I know and as I learn and develop even more I will share things with you such as recipes and ideas and new tips and techniques on the website at **http:/ /theultimatecellulitetreatment.com/**

For all your questions or to put your testimonial on the website simply email askbron@gmail.com.

Do keep in touch and do feel welcome to email me direct if you wish to converse with me or ask a question about *anything*.

One thing I want to do with this book is to not have it in some sort of order or method. Flick through and read whatever chapter takes your interest. It does not matter in what order you read the chapters, just enjoy and move your way through this book in whatever order takes your fancy.

Apply the methods, tips, techniques, and suggestions as you read and learn. But most of all enjoy.

Footnote: People have often told me over the years, and especially now for this book, that I should get before and after photos of my customers.

Firstly, I am yet to believe I have seen an authentic before and after photo.

In newspapers and magazines they usually use the same photo with alterations, such as zoom, shading and up or down lighting.

Not only did I not want to be tarred with that same brush of falsehood, but also, I find this practice humiliating for my ladies. Mostly I feel there is no need for evidence or reminders of what was, especially if it was unpleasant.

Get rid of your cellulite and put it out of your mind.

Forget the old you and rejoice in the new you.

"You must begin to think of yourself as becoming the person you want to be."

—David Viscott

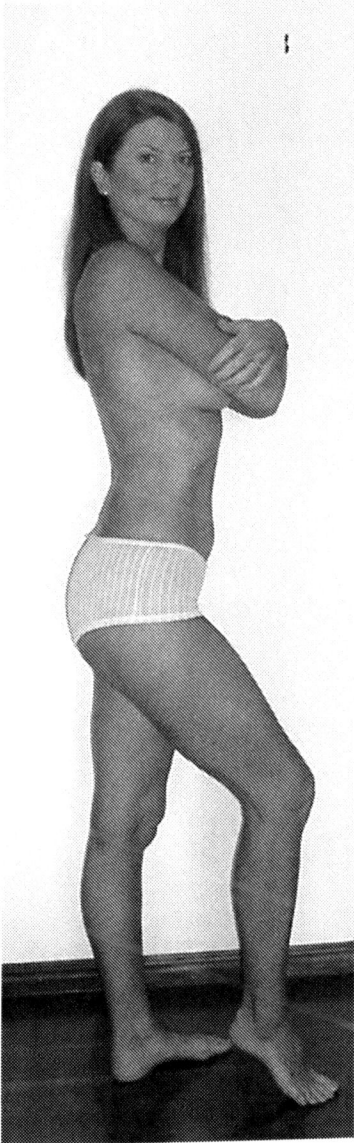

I had cellulite in my mid 20's and now I am 41, I got rid of it and it didn't come back. I have perfected my treatment and have treated women from all over Australia and this book now sells all over the world.

This photo has not been airbrushed or touched up in any way, it was taken by my friend Michelle with her husband's digital camera. In fact you can still see the picture hook on the wall from where we had removed the picture to get a blank wall in the background.

At the risk of appearing vain the point I am trying to make here with this photo is that the photo is completely natural as am I.

I am a bit lazy, I drink far too much wine according to my Mother and probably most Doctors and I've even been known to enjoy the odd cigar.

BUT I look like this because I eat well and do some little extra things that you will read about here in T.U.C.T. in a Book.

REASONS YOUR BODY STORES CELLULITE/ ENERGY

Specifically, you all have cellulite because you are not eliminating it–the waste, the additives, preservatives, and such that we consume.

This treatment is about getting all the parts of your body that contribute to eliminating waste working at their optimum levels to empty the rubbish tip.

I am not going to talk about diet or exercise, I will, although, talk about movement and what to eat and what not to eat later in this book.

So now
exercising = moving
dieti = food

When you refer to your '**diet**' you are referring to what you **do eat**, not what you do not.

Basic Body Types

To put it very, very simply, if you are storing most of your excess weight above your hips in your arms, breasts, hips and torso, with thinner legs, you are most likely **not eliminating properly and thoroughly**.

If you are holding most of your excess weight (stored energy) below your hips, mostly in your legs, hips, and thighs, then you most likely have a **sluggish circulation**.
So let's have a look at some simple things that will help.

The Stomach
–including chewing and helping your tummy digest.

Chewing your food is very, very important. Among other signals your body will produce juices in your mouth to help break down the food. This action of chewing really helps prepare the food to go into your stomach.

If the food has broken down substantially in your mouth, then there is less work for the stomach to do and therefore the food will spend less time in your stomach, so it moves through quickly and has no time to go off, producing yucky toxins.

When you chew your food, that chewing action sends messages to your stomach that food is coming and to prepare for it. Your body will close the pyloric sphincter to keep the food in your stomach. To close your pyloric sphincter intentionally you only need to chew on mouthful of food say one handful of nuts or a couple of olives.

Your stomach will produce juices to continue to break down the food you have chewed and contained.

If you have ever vomited then you will know that these stomach fluids are strong tasting and very acidic. And now your stomach has all the work to do; there aren't any teeth down there to chew and break down the foods ready for digestion.

So the less chewing you do in your mouth, the harder it is on your tummy. So **help your body by chewing your food properly**, which will also give your stomach the right messages to get ready for incoming stuff to digest.

Your Mother probably told you to chew your food properly as a child, as did her Mother and her Mother's Mother. They may not have known exactly why, but this is one of those many ol' wive's tales that we have been told for zillions of years, and we must continue the tradition.

I also recommend you do not drink water with food, especially a big meal at night as water can dilute those juices, making them less concentrated, and so it will take much longer for the foods to be broken down ready for your body to digest and metabolize.

Your Blood System.

It is important for your blood to be full of nutrients and oxygen and to be flowing freely (circulation). This is so that it can cart all the goodies around from the food you ate so that all your organs and all their cells are getting fed what they need, to work at their optimum levels. Great blood cleansers are natural foods. And as fresh as you can get your hands on is the best.

Apple cider vinegar and honey with hot water in the morning is the best blood cleanser I know, and is akin to eating an entire bowl of fruit for it's blood cleansing properties.

Real coffee brewed fresh is also a well known cleanser, oh, and there is always water which contains much oxygen.

An oft-forgotten source of oxygen is air, and your body will take in more if you breathe through your nose as opposed to your mouth. At rest, breathe deeply. Deep breathing warms the body and burns calories.

So to summarise:
I have read about so many different body shapes and what they mean and how to fix them, but really, basically there are three.

If you are **top heavy** then you need to concentrate on eliminating waste.

If you are **bottom heavy** then you need to concentrate on your circulation.

If you're retaining stored energy and are **heavy all over** then you need to concentrate your efforts on both.

This treatment will show you how to kick-start those areas that you need to help, and always keep in mind your weakness, be it circulation or elimination.

There are many other weaknesses that you may have. Mine is refined sugar, so I don't eat sweets, but I do eat good quality chocolate. And I would never go *near* cordial. I only drink the best coffee so that I don't need to add sugar.

If you enjoy a desert after dinner, try to replace sweets with a cheese platter some nights for a healthy refreshing change (tasty cheese and green apple are great together, and healthy). Add grapes, berries, and dried fruit for sweetness.

The sugars that are found in fruits and naturally sweet foods are good to eat. Our bodies are designed to handle and digest and to use these delicious sugars in their natural and original form.

We are simply not designed to digest/consume sugars that are refined and manufactured.

If you are a sucker for ice cream, try making your own from cream and condensed milk and fresh cream with frozen berries (it's all in the folding together of the ingredients). This way there are no added preservatives to keep it edible whilst being transported. Did you ever have homemade ice cream when you were a child? It is the best ice cream you'll ever taste.

Your weakness may be that you like salt and eat a lot of chips, or you like fried foods and eat a lot of battered foods. If you are in love with something, try to eat the best kind of that food that you can.

If you love a packet of chips for the saltiness, try to swap them for salted nuts and then downgrade to shelled peanuts.

When I get home, to fill the gap before dinner I eat olives, stuffed with feta or sun-dried tomatoes—salty and tasty, they can be very satisfying.

If you love fried and battered foods, go for a light Japanese Tempura-style batter, or crumb food with wholemeal bread-crumbs, and fry in a quality, light style of oil like grapeseed. You will find that grapeseed oil shallow fries really well.

Whatever you love to eat that you know is bad, try to eat a version of it that is healthier.

Tests have been done on hot chips for instance. The ones you buy frozen from the supermarket are generally healthier than the fast food outlet ones. So if you can't live without your hot chips, oven-bake them yourself and salt them with an alternative such as celery salt.

The great bonus is that once your body is cleaner it won't crave the salty and sugary flavours in the same way!

Anyway, I hope you get my drift and that you try to be honest with yourself, and try your hardest to always eat food that is as close to its natural state as possible.

Buy some herbs and experiment with them. You will find that there are many herbs that will give you that flavour hit that you crave. And always keep in mind your target area, whether it be circulation, elimination or both.

If you are ever in any doubt about what to eat email me at askbron@gmail.com.

TIPS AND TRICKS THAT WORK

I've called this chapter tips and tricks, as some of the things you can do are so easy and yet have so much effect it is like they are magic.

In this chapter you will learn some simple little things you can add to your life that will help you forever. You will also realise again that there is **no need for a diet** (the worst four letter word) or strenuous exercise or hard work.

Incorporating some or all off the suggestions in this book into your life will **enhance your life and lift your spirits** as well as your circulation, metabolism, and elimination.

The more tips you can take on, the better. If you do all the things I discuss in this book, your body should be functioning at its ultimate levels in no time at all.

How Long will this REALLY TAKE?

By this stage you may be wondering just how long this treatment will take. Firstly, I need you to get off the quick fix mindset such as a two week diet. This is not something that I can put a time on.

This treatment is not a temporary fix that will help you loose weight or cellulite so that after the treatment you wonder how long it will take for the weight to pile back on. Nothing could be further from the truth.

This is not a two or four week plan of doing everything completely different for a while so that you can get it over with and get back to your normal routine and hope that the weight takes its time coming back.

This is a change to the way you think about your body, and what you do with it.

This is NOT a diet nor is it an exercise routine.

This book discusses varied simple things that you can add to your life. **This is another reason why your cellulite won't come back**, as you will bring my principles into your life and hang onto them and use them always.

Although, I will say that when I am working with a client one on one, they will usually stay with me for about three months. In this time, much of their cellulite will move, and once it has started to move it will continue to flow and eliminate from their life, and then they are ok to go it alone.

From my experience with treating women over the last 15 years or so, the speed at which the cellulite moves is varied. I have given just one or two treatments and we both see an improvement. Whereas other women may not see a change for a month.

Generally within a month to six weeks you will see changes, from two to three months (I have seen it take 6 but rarely) your lumps and bumps will look worse as the cellulite breaks down.

At this stage you will do two things. 1. you will panic and probably email me then 2. you will rejoice because you are now on the downhill run girlfriend and can celebrate and relax.

When you reach this point it is very difficult to stop the cellulite on it's journey out of your body. Don't stop doing all the things you have learnt in your book but you can take it easy as all the hard work is now done.

But what do you do in ten years time?

I will also say that I am the first to admit that I might have a difficult six months or so, or have a bad year, and it gets to summer and I have a look at myself in a full-length mirror in my bikini, and I think *whoa, I have been a bit neglectful.*

This is when I realize I need to look at what I haven't been doing, and I will do a two week course of psyllium and start body brushing again. Just for a bit of a boost and a good cleanse. This may happen to you, too, but once you reapply all my principals again, your cellulite will soon move. If you are always eating well, eating real food, you shouldn't have any problems.

Try to always keep up the basics, ACV and honey in the morning, green tea after dinner, body brushing two or three times a week, and eat mostly natural foods.

It also doesn't matter how long you have had cellulite—2 months or 20 years—the reasons you have it are the same, and you need to turn your body around to get it functioning so that your body can eliminate waste and stored energy better.

OK, so let's have a look at some tips you can bring into your life that will get your body back working at its optimum levels, and you can be your ultimate self as soon as possible:

Psyllium Husks: Add psyllium husks to your diet NOW. They will clean all the undigested yucky stuff from your intestines small, large and bowels which is blocking parts of the lining that work to digest foods.

You want all of those miles of surface area to be clear to work. I have always advised that the psyllium husks can be taken at night before bed as they can slowly move through your intestines overnight, guaranteeing a regular movement every morning.

But if this doesn't suit you and you feel it would be better for YOU to have them in the morning, then do so; just take them, add them to your muesli. (Although I find they can bloat me slightly.)

Any health food shop, and these days most supermarkets, stock husks. Simply follow the instructions on the packet. There are many fibre drinks on the market that will gel up in water and cleanse you just like the psyllium husks. Basically they are all pretty good but as always, I like to go the most natural way possible rather than the imitation, and for intestinal cleansing the best and most natural are the husks. Do this for two weeks at a time and about every two to three months or so, or whenever you start feeling a little sluggish or bloated.

If you do buy an internal cleanser from you drug store or supermarket make sure that psyllium husks are at least listed as an ingredient.

Fasting/Detox: Detoxing is very popular lately and is very good for you. It is a great way to jump start your cleansing program, there are hundreds around and they're pretty much all good. **Even a one day detox, or a day or two of just fluids, will give your internal organs a much needed rest.**

A good detox can also help your stomach shrink back to its normal size if it has been stretched and takes too much food to fill you up. Your stomach is approximately 12 inches long and 6 inches wide with a capacity of approximately 1 quart, or just under 1 litre. Many of us put more than this into our stomachs every time we eat.

BUT, do read all the instructions that go with the Detox treatment and follow them. They are there for a reason. Do also consult a Doctor and get your essentials checked just to make sure you can handle it.

Very importantly, do not dive on in with all the enthusiasm you can muster straight into a two week detox. It is simply not safe or smart to suddenly starve yourself.

You can now get Detox Kits which are very effective that have nutrient supplements and helpful herbs and vitamins that you can take along with a sensible food plan. Otherwise, start with a two-day detox if it is your first time.

There are countless detox books available that outline several different durations or styles of detoxification, so find a nice easy short one and PLEASE do it on a weekend, or take a couple of days off work and really indulge in relaxation.

If you're not good at doing nothing, I can help you with that. Go out and buy a couple of books, a couple of those really expensive fashion magazines, a foot soak, nail buffer (battery-operated are more fun), a facial treatment, and why not a juicer and a heap of fruit. Empty the house, bolt the door, pull the phone out of the wall and have some 'Me Time'.

As you will learn when you read up on detoxifying, it is not necessarily a total denial of food or liquids, Some are liquid only for a couple of days with real (freshly squeezed) fruit juices. So treat yourself and get some tropical fruits and berries (berries are full of antioxidants), pop them in your zooza (processor) and make a fruit smoothie.

A mild detoxification might be to eat only fruit and veggies for four days—any more than that and your breath starts to smell and you'll stop getting invited to parties. Detoxifying is a great way to reduce the size of your stomach, plus it will give all your organs, especially the eliminatory ones, time to rest.

Chilli: carry dry chilli flakes or lecithin with you. Lecithin, like Chilli, acts as a fat metaboliser, meaning that it helps move fat smoothly through your body, helping you to eliminate it.

Close your sphincter: You must always close your sphincter (pyloric) before you drink alcohol due to its sugar content. See Do's and Don'ts for more details

Walk *before* eating, as opposed to after, if you have a choice. Studies have shown that your metabolism is increased during times of exercise AND most importantly that this increased rate of metabolism can last for a couple of hours after you have finished exercising. So eat during this time. Walking is very gentle and low intensity, so it is a very safe thing to do. Walking is good, and we actually do it a lot without realising it. If you find it a struggle at first to get out and about, please do not worry. Once you have started to eliminate some of the sludge, and your internals are getting nice and cleansed and are working better, the urge to move WILL COME TO YOU. So please don't force it—do the things I recommend and let the urge to move come to you.

Have Dry Skin Baths: After a shower, don't dry yourself. Let your skin do what it is designed to do, which is to dry by reacting with the air around you and creating its own moisturizers.

Learn How To Breathe: Breathing is very important; getting ultimate oxygen at every breath is very advantageous. Breathe through your nose. The air you breathe through your nose takes in more oxygen than your mouth. Plus the passage the air flows along when breathed through your nose will massage the frontal lobes of your brain. If you have children ensure that they always breathe through their noses. It's good for your brain and body especially in development years. Yoga can help you with this.

BE HAPPY: Happiness is healthiness. I'm serious, happy people are healthier and healthy people are happier (and not only because they can fit into their wedding dress). And it is easy to be happy. I'll tell you how.

Firstly, it is important to note that your subconscious mind does not know when you are lying or not. So even if you feel miserable, are highly stressed or feeling unwell, you can tell yourself the opposite. If I find myself consumed with worry over something, I say to myself, *everything will be great, it will all work out, no-one is going to die.*

If you find yourself feeling down (and we all have these days) help yourself by putting on a fake smile. Your brain doesn't know if your face is faking it or not, and studies on facial psychology have shown that by doing this the brain will think you are happy. And say "I feel GREAT, I am Happy" over and over, even if the first few times are through clenched teeth and a snarl. It really works. If you aren't good at this sort of thing or feel silly, put some signs up around the house, just simple little ones like:

- **I FEEL GREAT TODAY** ☺
- **Today will be a good day for me**
- **My Life is GOOD!**
- **I am HAPPY**

Paint them in happy colours. Get the kids to do them next school holiday. You will find that every time you walk past this sign you will read it subconsciously and therefore tell yourself that you feel great—and you will. Have you ever stood in the same lift or sat on the same toilet at work and read that same darn sign again and again and—ho hum—again and wondered why? It is just like a reflex; you automatically read the sign.

These signs are great for the whole family, and especially if you work in a negative environment, put up some signs and make if fun. Let your imagination run wild. Soon you will forget the signs are there, only reading them subconsciously but the message will still be getting through to your brain having the desired affect. Or influence.

If you are really interested in changing or improving your life dramatically I recommend you search for books and eBooks by Jeff Staniforth, Stuart Lichtman and Louise Hay for their invaluable teachings on affirmations.

Oh, and here is another big tip. Try to stop stressing about exercise. I'm sure that many of you have either given it a try and/or given up, or are exercising harder and harder and still not getting the results you want.

Remember replace the word ~~exercise~~ with **MOVEMENT**.
If you run out of milk–why not walk to the local shop for more.
Movement: OK, so everyone goes on about exercise and yes, it is so simple—energy in (food); energy out (exercise). But hey, for some of us exercising is yuck-O, embarrassing, or just too hard to get into. I understand completely.

People that exercise as part of their lives or routine find it difficult to understand why overweight people just don't get out and go for a run.

What they perhaps don't understand is that there is a HUGE gap between feeling bad about yourself, having no confidence, feeling depressed or scared, and being able to get up out of the chair and go to the gym. I do understand this.

Just getting started, being able to feel that you are capable of exercising can be a journey in itself. I do realize, I get it; I've been there. In fact I'm usually there at the start of every Spring.

If when you start out on the cellulite cleansing routine, you really, really don't feel like exercising, please don't, please don't force it. As you cleanse and encourage internal movement, you will find that as you feel lighter on your feet, less bloated and blocked, the interest and urge to move will come.

In the meantime, trick yourself into moving:

Parking your car: Don't we all just love to get that perfect car spot? The one that we always try for, when we go to our favourite shopping centre. The one that upsets us if someone else beats us to it! Next time you go to do your shopping, forget that favourite spot.

Park as far away from the entrance to the shopping centre as is safe. Park three our four rows away, park at the back where the shady trees are, you choose. You will find this to be much less stressful and it will force you to walk further, and always return your trolley. Therefore walking across the car park 4 times!

In a queue, stand on one foot at a time: Your body will be forced to try and balance you on one foot and use many muscles to do so, burning up calories in the process. You only need to lift your foot half an inch–keep it subtle in public.

Socialise on your feet:
When at a bar out for a drink, always stand–burns more calories. So if you enjoy a drink with your friends, do so without the guilt. Whilst on a serious cleanse, red wine is best. Lowest sugar, and high in the good stuff, as the good stuff is in the skin of the grape. Mind you, there are white wines coming out that include the skins, but they are far and few between, but stay tuned on that one. Oh, and dance.

Coffee and Cake: If you crave a coffee and some killer chocolate cake, find a café you like located near a park–walk the park and then **have your cake AND EAT IT TOO! WITH NO GUILT!** Woo Hooo; you will feel great. See how easy this can be?!

Always Stand Whilst On Public Transport: if you travel by train, one hour each way to and from work use this time. This is serious exercise if you are standing for two hours a day. Remember to alternate legs. Balancing core muscles and the movement of the vehicle will only help. Breathe deeply through your nose and rhythmic, this will help warm your body and burn calories.

Which Exercise Is Best For Me?

Please don't worry about which exercise is the best one for you to do. Get every DVD or video you can lay your hands on. Borrow from your friends and even swap. I have Pilates, fit ball DVD's, Oxercise, you name it. To be honest, I've got ones I haven't even watched yet and yes, I have sat on the couch and watched one, just to check it out and make sure it is a good quality video! There is something delightfully naughty about watching an exercise video whilst eating chocolate!

Mostly, I haven't made it to the advanced levels, some of you will, some of you won't—who cares? It doesn't matter. If you have a variation of DVD's you can do a Pilates workout if you feel like it or go outside for a walk if it is a lovely day. It is good to have options.

But between you and me, if you only want to get one DVD, then get a Pilates one. It is one of the more simple workouts to do but the results are incredible. I can tell you that if you do Pilates three times one week, then three times the next week, you will already notice a big improvement in how you do the Pilates movements in that second week. In the third week you will notice that you even walk differently, steady and strong, but graceful. You will tend to glide along more. Seriously! If you want to talk to me about which Pilates to do, drop me a line and we can have a chat.

I don't know if blonde girls have more fun but I do know that Pilates' girls do!

If you don't live in an area near a park or the beach, drive to one and then go for a walk. Go to the most expensive suburb within your reach and walk along the beautiful tree lined streets, look at all the houses as you stride by and dream to your heart's content. Why not? You can walk anywhere you want to.

There are many activities that you may want to do once you start feeling light on your feet–just don't force it. Join a dance lesson club or (and this is great) join a lawn bowls club. If you have never played lawn bowls, go to a social game and you will be amazed at how much your bottom (lower glutes) will hurt in two days' time. So if you have a saggy bottom–go bowling. Or try something different like pole dancing! I even have a pedal machine that I can sit on the couch and peddle. My friends laugh at me sitting on the lounge watching a movie with a glass of wine in one hand and the remote in the other whilst quietly peddling away.

Watch Your Stress Levels: Stress creates a fluid called adrenaline and other chemicals such as cortisol and epinephrine hormones, which are the "Fight or Flight" response we all have when put under increased STRESS. If this fluid is not used it will be stored somewhere as waste–not good.

If you are stressed, then you definitely need to add movement to your life.

Oh, and no matter what is causing your stress, always ask yourself, is there anything I can do, say, or act upon to change what is causing my stress? If the answer is yes, then you owe it to yourself to take that action; act now, do not procrastinate, even if what you do turns out to be wrong–at least you acted with your best of intentions.

If things are really extreme ask yourself *will anyone die?* If the answer is yes–then take some action fast! Do what you can and then move on. If the answer is no, then for your body's sake **let the problem go**. STOP thinking about it, escape from the thoughts revolving around your head—go see a movie, or sink yourself into a good book.

Drink Shower Water: Warm water is wonderful for flushing the kidneys and liver, plus it makes the whites of your eyes especially white and clear. So drink the warm water in the shower three or four big gulps will do you wonders.

Drink Green Tea: Green tea is a wonderful aid for digestion. If you drink green tea on an empty stomach it will cleanse. If you drink it after a meal it will greatly aid your digestion. If you find the taste unsavoury just add a squeeze of lemon.

Also Finish Your Shower With A Cold Blast: You will feel your skin react and tighten–you may also gasp and scream as I do–but this is sooo good for awakening your skin as an eliminatory organ, reminding the skin that it can move and tighten and relax and eliminate. And you will feel it do it!

THE TOP TEN DO'S AND DON'TS

Do's

1. **Drink Apple Cider and Honey**

2. **Body Brush**

3. **Take psyllium husks**

4. **Take Lecithin or eat chilli**

5. **Take vitamin supplements**

6. **Drink Water**

7. **Get yourself a Fit Ball**

8. **Close your sphincter**

9. **Eat Real Food**

10. **Stretch & Move**

Explanations:

#1. APPLE CIDER VINEGAR & HONEY

Drink apple cider vinegar and honey (ACV & H) every morning whether you are cleansing or not. It is the best way to start the day.

Honey is packed full of antioxidants. There has been a lot of talk about antioxidants; we have been told by the medical experts that they are good for us but sometimes we forget why, because when we read about them it can seem so complicated that it is easy to forget. So I am going to tell you about antioxidants in a way that I understand them that should help you too.

Let's start with a simple ABC

A.   Cells consist of molecules.

B.   Molecules consist of atoms.

C.   Atoms consist of a nucleus, neutrons, protons, and **electrons**.

OK, so far so good.

Now, electrons are required to keep the atom stable. If the atom doesn't have enough of their own electrons, they will actually share electrons with other atoms. (Isn't that sweet?)

To share the electrons, atoms don't split electrons in half, but bond themselves together, enabling them to literally share electrons to ensure they maintain stability.

If this bond is weak and splits it becomes a Free Radical which is a loose or unbalanced atom or molecule.

Free radicals will attack the nearest unstable atom to steal it's electron, thereby turning that atom into a free radical as well, and so on it goes, and eventually this vicious cycle will destroy the entire living cell.

Not all free radicals are bad, though. Free radicals are sometimes created by our body's immune system to fight bacteria and viruses. But sometimes they are spawned from pollution, radiation, cigarette smoke, and herbicides.

Antioxidants can stop the free radicals from stealing electrons from other atoms, as they are able to donate to the atoms one of their own electrons. They are little sweet, too. Ironically, often antioxidant-containing foods are sweet, such as berries and honey.

So now I hope you understand a little better that we need to always have antioxidants available within our systems to supply electrons to atoms (when they are needed to stabilise atoms) and in turn keeping your cells alive.

An example of an essential time to have available antioxidants is after you've had a virus such as the flu. Your body would have been producing free radicals to fight the virus (bad cells) so you now would require antioxidants to repair the good cells.

Regularly consuming honey, such as drinking apple cider and vinegar every morning, will maintain healthy levels of antioxidants in your blood.

The combination of the apple cider, honey, and warm water cleanses your blood. The cleansing and antibiotic properties are equal to eating a bowl of fruit, and the warm water helps to carry it through your system to purify your blood, reduce fat, and clean your bowels. It really is a fabulous all-in-one. If you can't drink the apple cider vinegar, swap it for lemon juice. Or better yet, take ACV tablets instead. If you health food shop doesn't stock them yet, ask them to.

1 soup spoon Apple Cider Vinegar

1 soup spoon Honey

Top up cup with hot water

Green Tea is also one of the best ways to get your supply of antioxidants. Green Tea has so impressed health professionals around the world with it's effective antioxidants that neutralise free radicals that you will soon hear about the effectiveness of green tea against cancer. And not only is that impressive but White Tea is showing itself to be even more effective than green tea although caffeine levels are higher but thankfully both are available in caffeine free varieties. When choosing caffeine free products select the one that states it is 'naturally decaffeinated'.

Everyone I meet that drinks green tea seems to be very healthy and always mention that they drink the tea. I have a friend who has drank green tea most of her life, morning and night and she has never ever had cellulite–and at her age she now never will.

#2 BODY BRUSH

Body brushing is such an essential part of this treatment I have dedicated an entire chapter to it. So get yourself a cactus or natural fibre brush as soon as possible. It must be a stiff, natural fibre brush, and it may take you a little while to get used to. If you do experience difficulties getting the right brush in your part of the world please contact me and I will get one to you.

#3 PSYLLIUM HUSKS

Psyllium husks are a soluble fibre in its purest form. To take, add two teaspoons of psyllium husks to water, stir, and drink. You must drink it straightaway as the little seeds swell up in water and gel. You want this gel to form in your stomach, not in the glass.

This psyllium gel moves slowly through your intestines, stimulating the transport of waste. The resulting bulk stimulates a reflex contraction of the walls of the bowel. This is great exercise for the intestinal walls and will encourage your eliminatory organs to move waste through the system with greater efficiency. This is good to do several times a year. Do it at the start of every season.

Take the psyllium husks at night before you go to bed. As you may bloat slightly from them at first. Take them for two weeks; you don't want to take them for long periods of time. Take them for two weeks every three months. The easiest way is to pop a teaspoon of husks into a wide tumbler, swirl them around like mad, and then gulp down as swiftly as possible. You'll need to refill the glass to get them all down and rinse your mouth. You can also get them in capsule form and is the easiest way to take them.

#4 CHILLI:

The **great fat metaboliser**. Chilli metabolises fats whilst in your stomach. So add chilli to everything and it will help you no end. I LOVE eating cheese and biscuits (with a glass of wine), so I always add chilli to my antipasto platters. Shake on some dry chilli flakes or make your own chilli paste by crushing fresh ones in your zooza with some grapeseed oil. If you buy nuts, get the chilli flavoured ones, same with everything. Chilli is very cheap, and if the label says there is chilli in the product, then the ingredients will confirm.

Lecithin is also brilliant at dealing with fats if you don't like the side effects of chilli (heat at both ends). This is great news if you can't handle the heat of the chilli. Lecithin has many nicknames such as the 'fat grabber', but mostly is known as a fat emulsifier. The alternative industry belief is that lecithin will eliminate the fatty foods that you eat whilst it is in your tummy. Also, if you eat a low or non-fat meal, the lecithin will enter your system and work on eliminating the hard core fat that sits under your skin. It is also wonderful for your brain, and in fact, every cell in your body.

#5 VITAMINS:

It is really important to get all the vitamins your body requires for normal cellular function. Just imagine if every single cell in your body is functioning to its ultimate best because they are getting all their required vitamins and nutrients. Do get with a program so that all your vitamins are the same brand, and all-natural. If you get an organized package each month, then you know you are getting all your vitamins balanced correctly and delivered each month.

I take vitamins every day and I have my favourites, of course. Make sure you get ones that are free of preservatives. Many vitamin tablets have preservatives in them to keep their shape. I have taken vitamins in pill form and liquid form and now also the oral spray. Just get the ones that suit you. If the pills make you feel like a giant baby rattle then perhaps the liquid variety are better suited for your needs. If you want to know where I get my vitamins, drop me an email and I can advise you personally what you may need. I love the liquid vitamins, and you can get some that taste great. I add mine to champagne to make a yummy and oh-so-healthy Champagne cocktail!

Vitamins are especially important if you can't shop for fresh food daily. Unfortunately, most of us get our produce from a supermarket, so it is not fresh. Michael Montignac's book *The Montignac Method* explains frighteningly clearly the rapid reduction of vitamin content in foods as the days, hours, and minutes go by, especially if they have been pre-cut and packaged for your convenience.

#6 WATER:

60 to 70 % of us is water–don't let this get low, as every single cell requires water. But don't freak out too much and go to extremes. Get into the habit of carrying a 500 ml bottle around with you and continually sip all day, rather than try to guzzle a couple of glasses when you remember. If you sip all day and fill up the bottle two to three times a day, you are doing great.

But this, of course, depends on your daily activity. If you work outdoors doing physical work, you could require five litres per day.

Try different things, like squeezing a lemon or orange into the water, or drink herbal tea. If you have tried herbal tea and it made your face screw up like never before, please don't be so disenchanted as to give it up. Best thing to do is to go and get singular bags of all types of herbal tea and try them one by one. I add honey to most of them. Honey is antibacterial and is a wonderful healthy sweetener.

#7 FIT BALL:

When you sit on a ball you are exercising because your body needs to balance. Balancing uses a lot of muscles. Building muscle strength is good, as your body uses more calories for muscle cells than it does for your stored fat cells.

It is really great for you to sit on whilst watching TV or knitting or even reading a magazine. To choose your size, when you sit on it, your knees should be at a right angle to the floor. Always sit up straight on the ball, and get yourself a basic video that will teach you fit ball posture. This is extremely important to get maximum benefit. Just think, you can watch the midday movie and not feel guilty about it, because you are using your stored energy. If you do nothing else, no exercise at all whatsoever, then get yourself a fit ball and sit yourself down.

8 CLOSE YOUR SPHINCTER:

Not that sphincter! There is another one. On the way from your stomach to your intestine is the pyloric sphincter. The pyloric sphincter is a ring of muscle that creates a gate between your stomach and small intestine. When you begin to eat food, the chewing action sends off a stream of messages around your body. These alert certain parts to prepare for food. **One of these messages tells the stomach sphincter to close** so that the stomach can contain the food in one area so as to break it down to use around the body.

If you have a drink, the fluid will rush straight through to your intestines. If this is a particularly sugary drink such as cola or alcohol, the sugars will go straight through without being properly digested and converted into the correct sugars for the body. Therefore, it is extremely important to close this sphincter before you have a glass of wine.

To close your sphincter therefore all you need to do is chew some food. One handful of nuts or even three olives will do it.

We are finally starting to see low sugar, low calorie, and 'light' drinks for women, but they have been a long time coming, and there aren't many. If I am drinking during the day, I weaken the sugar (and therefore alcohol content) of the wine by making a spritzer.

Australia is famous for their barbeques, but unless you drink beer, there are very few alternatives to drinking full-strength drinks. Half wine and half mineral water with a dash of liquid vitamins or a squirt of lemon or lime juice is a great alternative.

If you are out for a drink after work and realize that you haven't eaten since lunch time, you need to eat. Most bars have nuts–better than chips. Just know that a packet of cashews, albeit high in fat, is much better than drinking with your sphincter open. **You don't need to eat much; the chewing action is important**, not the amount of food. **One bickie with cheese will do it, one dolmade, five peanuts or three olives will do it**, too. Get the nuts with the skins on–the skins are high in iron. But you'll need to laugh with your hand over your mouth until you have been to the bathroom to check your teeth for skins, like you do with cracked pepper.

If you are serious about cleansing but do live a social life style, it may be a good idea to keep a packet of nuts or seeds or even sultanas in your purse or glove compartment of your car.

**Or my personal favourite sphincter closer:
Order a Martini and eat the olive first!**

#9 EAT REAL FOOD & CHOCOLATE

Our bodies were not designed to eat anything other than real food. By real food I mean food that is in its natural state. We were not designed to consume additives or preservatives or chemicals of any kind. So eat food as close to its natural form as possible.

You will read more about this in the chapter *Eat Food*.

If you want to eat chocolate, for instance, eat good quality chocolate. Some people even report that chocolate is good for you.

The better the quality—the purer the chocolate. Plus it is such a happy food that it can bring on feelings of joy–I'm serious.

Chocolate is not bad for you–if you are eating well and taking supplements, then your body will not need to keep the sugars from the chocolate for energy as it will already have plenty from the healthy foods you eat and the vitamins you take.

Yep, you can have your cake and eat it too.
In fact, I eat chocolate almost every day.

#10 STRETCH & MOVE

Stretching your muscles is extremely good for you and will enhance your physical fitness in the most gentle way. Stretch in the morning before you get out of bed. Just do small stretches to every part of your body whilst the muscles are still warm from your sleep. Start by flexing your feet forward and back and hold the stretch for a breath or three.

Don'ts

1. **Diet**

2. **Eat White flour**

3. **Potatoes**

4. **Bananas**

5. **Smoke mass produced cigarettes**

6. **Drink fizzy/soft drinks (Champagne excluded)**

7. **Drink water with meals**

8. **Refer to your stored/unused energy as fat**

9. **Weigh yourself every day**

10. **Stress**

Explanations:

#1. DIET

There are **three major reasons why you should not diet,** not even reduce the amount of food you eat.

Reason One: Your body has an inbuilt monitor that keeps your weight steady. For instance if you weigh 80 kg's and have done for more than a year, your body will assume that this is the weight it should be.

If you suddenly semi-starve yourself to lose the weight, this monitor will tell the body to start storing energy to keep your weight steady, so when you diet, **your body will actually work against you.**

Reason Two: As soon as you stop starving yourself, your body will try to keep and store everything it can. This is why your weight can quickly increase after a diet to get it back up to that 80 kg's.

When you finish your diet, you actually put on more weight than you were originally, and you will now find yourself six months later to be 5 kg's heavier.

Reason Three: You could be the same weight after a diet, but you will have more fat content than you did before. **When you diet, you loose fat and muscle weight**. This is very bad, as muscle burns more calories.

The higher your muscle content, the higher the usage of energy. **Ten pounds of muscle will burn 500 calories per day** just sitting around. So if you loose this much muscle, you need to **consume 500 less calories per day to keep your weight down.**

This is where dieters end up in a downward spiral of eating less and less and less to loose weight. When the diet is over and normal eating habits return, you gain weight again and none of it is muscle; it is all fat.

So you need to be eating 500 to 1000 calories less per day than you did before the diet. So please don't diet. Think quality of food, not quantity. And think about getting leg and wrist band weights for when you walk, or better still, pump some iron to build up your muscle content. If you have kids, don't just supervise their play, play with them. Even thumb wrestling is exercise–especially if you are sitting on fit balls. If you are over 40, you probably should look at increasing your muscle content.

So please PLEASE, don't stop eating, DO NOT DIET just change what you eat. Make sure everything or at least most of what you put in your mouth is real. If it didn't exist in our diet 100 years ago, then you shouldn't eat it now. Save the modern food for special occasions and when you go out.

#2. WHITE FLOUR:

Ever eaten white flour and felt it stick to your teeth?
White flour clogs up your system and has only recently been part of our diets. Some factions of thought lay the blame for cellulite totally with the consumption of white flour. When first introduced, it was only eaten by the extremely wealthy or Royal few–hence they started getting fat. Think of all those old portraits of Royal families in your history books, they were always huge and in many cultures around the world overweight people are still assumed to be wealthy. Then the processing became cheaper and we can all afford it, and we are all getting fat now. If you must, try to at least get white with bran

included. This will help move the white flour through your body.

But preferably eat bread made from stone-ground whole meal flour. You can even get bread with psyllium husks in it! When you pick up real bread it feels much heavier than standard bread, twice as heavy. It will also fill you up more so you will find that you will eat less real bread than you did eating white bread.

If you love your white bread, just persevere. You will get used to the whole meal bread. I have converted many. Plus, wholemeal bread fills you up more. You'll go from two white bread sandwiches down to one wholemeal one. That equals less butter and fewer fillings.

Also try to avoid yeast and 'raising agents' in biscuits, as they work by generating bubbles of carbon dioxide gas that become trapped inside the mixture and inflate it.

If this process is not complete when you consume a product, it will complete its process in your stomach. Your stomach is not designed to cope with this. Bread-raising must be complete when you eat the food. There are even some bread makers and pizza dough makers who are mindful to this process and completely raise the dough before it is cooked so that the 'raising' will not occur in your tummy.

#3. POTATOES

Potatoes are full of bad carbohydrates and starch, besides, until recently, potatoes were only fed to pigs. Yes, potatoes are pig food and should remain as such. What do farmers particularly want pigs to do? Get fat fast! So limit them or give them up all together, especially whilst on a cleansing or weight loss programme.

#4. BANANAS

Bananas are fine if you are a child, athlete or monkey. Yes, bananas are also meant for animals–monkeys. Or, as I have recently discovered—pregnant. Bananas are very high in energy. Monkeys are constantly on the move, swinging around trees. Even at rest, they are fidgeting and preening each other, so they never really keep still and they need and more importantly use the energy they get from bananas. Children are the same, so they will have no troubles burning the energy they get from eating bananas. So unless you are confident that you are going to burn this energy, leave them well alone.

#5. SMOKING:

Every single cigarette contains THOUSANDS of toxins. YUCK. We are trying to get rid of the toxins not make more. If you must smoke whilst on a cleanse, get raw tobacco or a decent cigar instead. Or of you really *need* the release of the deep breath then go herbal.

#6. FIZZY DRINKS

Seriously, no explanation is required–just read the ingredients. Or complete the second sentence:

1. Orange juice is made from oranges.

2. Cola/Soda is made from….?

N.B. Champagne is made from grapes, grapes are fruit and fruit is good for you. Champagne is allowed.

#7. DRINK WATER WITH MEALS

Water can dilute your gastric juices and will therefore slow down metabolism in the stomach. Drink water only half an hour before and after finishing a meal. If you eat three or four times a day and have a glass of water half an hour before and afterwards, you are drinking plenty of water. If you eat three meals a day with a morning and afternoon snack, and you drink one glass of water before and after you eat, that equals 10 glasses of water. This is plenty and perfect.

#8. REFER TO STORED ENERGY AS FAT

Fat is an ugly three letter word, stop using it. Don't call yourself or your friends' fat. You and they simply have too much energy stored for reasons that are not anyone's fault.

#9. WEIGH YOURSELF EVERY DAY

Our weight fluctuates from day to day, even within one day and it can be quite disheartening to see you've gained a kilo when you have been so good. This can be especially worse at 'that' time of the month.

Also, if you are exercising and gaining muscle weight, you may be loosing inches but gaining pounds at the same time because muscle is much heavier than fat. Think of the fat around your steak. A Piece of fat is much lighter than the same size of meat.

If you are wanting to lose weight, try to keep from weighing yourself every day, but try to leave it to a couple of times a month or not at all, not ever, in fact never! Shocking I know. It is not so much about how much you weigh, but how toned you are, if you fit into your favourite dress again, AND HOW YOU FEEL.

If you must weigh yourself at all, do it first thing in the morning, after you have been to the toilet, before you drink, before you even think, before you eat.

You should be at your lowest weight then and this is therefore much more motivating.

#10. STRESS

Stress creates a fluid called adrenaline. If this fluid is not used, it will be stored somewhere as waste—not good. If you are stressed, then you definitely need to add movement to your life. Affirmations can be a wonderful help for your stress.

"The future is something which everyone reaches at the rate of sixty minutes an hour,
whatever she does, whoever she is."

—C. S. Lewis

EAT FOOD

OK, so here's a news flash for you girls out there–
FOOD IS GOOD FOR YOU. EAT IT.

Yes, I can promise you that. So I want you to get into the mind set that eating is good and enjoyable and will make you feel good in mind, body, and spirit. We've been doing it for thousands upon thousands of years and it never hurt anyone yet. But in the last few hundred years, for the first time, we are seeing a lot of overweight people. And it is mostly due to what we ate then compared to what we eat now.

I am a great fan of food, and encourage you all to get back to enjoying food, having dinner parties, and making food your friend again.

Mind you, what you eat must be good food, and it is very, very easy to recognize the good from the bad. Here are some things that you need to start doing straight away.

***Shop mostly from the walls,
not the aisles of your supermarket.***

Most of the items in the aisles are not real foods. But the walls contain your vegetable department, dairy, and the delicatessen–all fresh foods. I personally only shop for fresh food if possible at the local green grocer, as their produce hasn't been all over the country in trucks, often getting to the supermarket already at the very least a week old. All the rest of my shopping is done online with a global service that works even in regional areas where I live. I never have to lug home piles of toilet rolls, heavy cleaning products, or even a broom any more. No stress.

I want you to start reading the ingredients on EVERY item *before* you put it in your trolley. Don't eat anything with numbers on it, or preservatives, colours, flavours, or any kind of additive. Even with the simplest of foods, you will be amazed when you read the ingredients. Beware of low fat, low carb and low salt products. Often the process that foods go through to remove fat or salt is a chemical one, and will leave traces in its wake for you to consume.

The low salt butter in my fridge says it contains milk solids, water, and salt. I get the low salt, as the salt in butter is to help it keep. These days we all have a fridge, so you don't need that high salt content. If you have a tub of butter or margarine that has more ingredients than three or four, get rid of it, because that is what butter is: milk solids, water, and salt. Keep this in mind with all Dairy products/milk products. And they are an essential part of any good food plan especially yoghurt which is full of the good bacterias.

Go through your kitchen and box up all those packets of stuff–dried or canned or any food that has numbers, preservatives, or colours added, and throw it out. Don't worry too much about sugar or salt; they are not bad for you. Michael Montignac is the absolute guru on this–do get his book and read it.

Do keep in mind that toasted cereals are coated in copious amounts of sugar. Toast anything–a piece of bread even and once toasted the flavour becomes more savoury. To combat this and to make the cereal sweet too many sugars or worse sweeteners are added.

If you have toasted breakfast cereal in your cupboard REGARDLESS of all the good things it says it has in it such as fibre and fruit—remove it from your life or finish it and don't buy any more, at least whilst you are on this cleanse or trying to lessen your stored energy.

Dr. Phil McGraw talks extensively about a "fail-safe environment"–he is sooo right. Get his book too, if you are wanting to loose weight as well as your cellulite. A fail-safe environment means that you remove all the things that you should not eat from your home. This way, when you are hungry, the only options you have to eat at home are good healthy ones.

Back to basics is the way I want you to think as far as food goes. All you have to realize is that our bodies were created to eat and utilize certain foods for normal bodily functions to

operate. Our bodies were not designed to process or metabolize anything fake.

**Think back a hundred years–if we didn't eat it then,
don't eat it now.**

Our bodies were not designed to eat preservatives or colorants
or flavour enhancers or thickeners (salad dressings are full of
them—make your own at home, ask me or any European or
from an old country how if you're not sure) and all those
numbers that come out of a laboratory, not out of the ground.
These are the things that really clog up our systems. They
block normal processing such as metabolism and eliminating
waste, which are ESSENTIAL for staying healthy and to prevent your body from over storing energy. I have it on good
authority that there are food scientists trying to do the right
thing, and are using natural preservatives more and more
where they can.

Try to make your staple diet raw food as opposed to pasta or
bread. Salads are great and soups are also as the vitamins are
contained in the liquid the vegetables are cooked in. When
you reach for a snack in the fridge grab an apple or a bunch of
grapes (add a dob of honey for a taste sensation, the Israelis do
it for a treat on New Years Eve) or a stick of celery or carrot
(dip into a homemade dip–tuna, soya mayo, chilli and lemon
grass).

And remember, stop calling your excess weight FAT. It is simply stored energy that hasn't been used or cannot be elimi-

nated due to blocked eliminatory organs or slow metabolism, circulation or all of the above.

And while I'm on the subject of stored energy, don't worry so much about so-called fat contents of food. A good example is the humble avocado. Avocado is almost a staple food for me and I happily indulge daily when they're in season.

Avocadoes are notoriously high in fat BUT they are not actually that high in fat at all and more importantly they are easily digested, very high in mineral and vitamin content, and contain potassium, magnesium, folate, dietary fibre, riboflavin, and vitamins C, E, and B6.

Oh, and they actually only contain about 5 grams of fat anyway, and only twenty calories.

Importantly, they are also a very soft food, not complex, and are therefore very easy for the body to breakdown and digest.

This is an extremely important thing to remember–always consider the digestibility of foods. The avocado will move through your body at rapid speeds, as it is soft and easy to break down.

The faster food moves through you, the better. And when you eat avocados, don't be stingy, don't hold back. I will have half an Avocado on one piece of toast with real butter and cracked pepper–yum, yum–great for breakfast, lunch, or a snack;

topped with alfalfa sprouts is sooo good for you. To keep the other half fresh, use the half that doesn't hold the stone first, then put the halves together the empty half and the half with the stone and foil them up together and that stone will keep it fresh much longer.

An example of a harder food would be red meat. Just looking at a steak you can see the weight and the solidness, and now picture all your little enzymes and things in your tummy trying to break it down. Not an easy task. DO NOT misinterpret this to mean that steak is bad—it is not. Red meat is wonderful and if you look back in time–all the way back to our primitive days–all we ate was meat and fruit and berries.

Our body is perfectly designed to eat and digest such things, so continue to enjoy that T-Bone or that delicious Porterhouse or Scotch Fillet steak. Just remember to chew it well so your tummy has less work to do.

If you find a bit of meat is difficult to chew, don't swallow it for your tummy to sort out later, spit it out. If your teeth can't break it down don't expect your stomach to. If you're out, pop it into your napkin as discretely as possible and then ask the waiter for a new one.

But I will say when you first start eating well, leave eating heavy food such as red meat to only a couple of times a week and ALWAYS have that heavy meal as early in the evening as possible, OR even better, have your steak meals at lunch time.

Also, you can help by getting some living enzymes into your tummy at the same time as you eat the steak. This is done by having your steak with a salad that includes alfalfa sprouts. These alfalfa sprouts are alive when you eat them and will really help your body break down heavy solid foods to move everything through the body as soon as possible. Get a sprout farm.

Meat balls are a good way to eat red meat, as you can add veggies in them and you can coat them in psyllium husks to help absorb any extra moisture to help you roll them.

What comes in must come out!

When your poo smells a little like your last meal because it is still that fresh, then you will know that your metabolism is moving and grooving as fast as it should be. Sorry to mention the poo word; but whilst I'm here on the subject I may as well take this opportunity to talk about it. Poo is very important—for obvious reasons, if you're not pooing regularly, this is may be a clue that you have a sluggish bowel or digestive system. If this is the case, you need to concentrate on that area. You will need to look at increasing your fibre intake, and psyllium husks are an easy way to do this.

I want all of you to—as gross as this may be for you (just don't tell anyone) but I want you to look at your poo every time you go. It should be light in colour and light in weight and may even float.

At first when you start cleansing this won't necessarily be the case and you will likely get two-toned ones as you cleanse out old waste. This is good; don't worry. The darker the poo, the older it is. If all your poos are dark, then keep adding more fibre to your diet to get the food moving quicker.

Remember, there is a lot of fibre in fruit and vegetables, especially dark leafy veggies. Always keep in mind what you are aiming for, and that is nice light floaty ones every day. You'll giggle to yourself as you skip out of the toilet with an inner smile on your face when you've just done a good one!

This steady movement of food is very important and really easy to understand. When you buy a steak or chicken or fish or anything fresh, and you bring him home–where do you keep him until you are ready to prepare the meal? On the front porch? In the lounge, on the coffee table, or on the kitchen bench? Definitely not, you pop him straight into the fridge and bring him out at the last possible moment for cooking. Why? Well to keep him all fresh and lovely, of course. So you wouldn't keep fresh food anywhere other than the fridge, and you certainly wouldn't keep it in a hot place, say, somewhere wet and usually around 37 degrees hot. Such as your stomach.

So now imagine your tummy, which is an environment I just described. If you put meat in your tummy and let it sit there for several hours, what sort of condition would it be in–would it then be edible? I think not.

It is important for your digestive and metabolism systems, and more importantly your eliminatory systems, to be working at their ultimate levels to get that steak moving through the system as quickly and as efficiently as possible.

If meat isn't refrigerated, it goes off. If it goes off in your stomach, it will create bad toxins, which your body will not eliminate very efficiently. Knowing this and knowing how good meat is for you, just remember to always help it through. You can do this by eating smaller portions, with some living enzymes, and also by eating it earlier in the day so your body is awake and busy when it is being metabolized. Also, the less cooked, the easier it is to digest. A steak cooked 'well done' is much harder or firmer than a rare cooked steak.

Another way to help digestion is by doing some light exercise before a heavy or any meal. It is well documented that exercise, even very light exercise such as walking, not only increases your metabolic rate but also keeps it at a higher level for some time after you have finished exercising.

If you have kids ask them to find out what we used to eat in the Stone Age or even in the Medieval Age as a little holiday project. Not that long ago, only monkeys ate bananas and pigs ate potatoes; we did not–keep this in mind and keep them to a minimum.

Eating out? Always eat the specials at restaurants, as they contain the freshest ingredients. Not only are they fresh, but just as importantly, the specials are what the chef is excited about and will put his heart into, as he is probably excited about the main ingredient which he got in fresh that morning, opposed to the everyday menu meals that are churned out without as much love.

Oh, and add chilli to everything. If you eat chilli, you will rarely get a cold even when the entire office has the latest allergy, as it is so high in vitamin C. It also aids metabolism and helps eliminate fat in foods whilst it is still in your tummy so that your body doesn't keep it. Lecithin does the same thing.

If you can't eat chilli, pop a lecithin capsule every time you eat some fatty foods. Oh, and if you ever over chilli yourself as I manage to do ALL THE TIME, don't drink water, you need dairy–it acts as a coolant. Milk is the easiest, or cheese. For an extremely hot mouth, take a mouthful of milk and hold it in your mouth for half a minute; two or three times should do it. If you rub chilli on your skin by accident, put some milk on a paper towel and dab it on the burn.

OK, some more food tips for you …

Eating by Colours

I know it can be very difficult to know what food is good for you and which ones to eat and how to ensure that you and **your family are getting a good cross section of vitamins** from the food you serve them.

The easiest way to do this is to eat by colours.

Different coloured foods contain different types of vitamins and nutrients.

Most restaurants and cafes offer a 'green' salad, and they are fine and trendy, but all those leafy green veggies contain similar vitamins, so you wouldn't want to only eat green salads all the time.

When you shop for vegetables get different coloured ones. For a roast, if you have pumpkin (orange); squash (yellow); onion or garlic (white), beans or peas (green), and capsicum you have such a clear difference of colours, and can therefore be assured that you are getting a good variety of vitamins as well. The same theory goes for casseroles, soups and salads. So when you go to the grocers, fill your basket with as many different colours as you can. Also note the vitamin content of light and dark green leafy vegetables differ.

Apple Cider Vinegar

Apple cider vinegar, honey, and hot water are another way of cleansing your blood. I can't tell you how many people I have treated who say "oh my great Grand Mother used to drink that!" or similar. This is another wonderful tip for cleansing that we used to drink years gone by, but somehow we have forgotten. A soup spoon of vinegar, then a soup spoon of honey into a mug, then top with hot water. Always drink first thing in the morning. It may take you a little while to get used to the taste; use extra honey until you do. Most people cannot go back to a coffee in the morning, "it just seems too heavy", is what they usually say. If you really can't stomach the ACV + Honey drink you can get the ACV in tablet form. Check with your Drug Store.

Your body does its natural body cleansing in the morning, so help it along by eating fruit. Any fruit is great. Apples, of course, and berries, but if time-consumed and you only have time for one piece of fruit, make it a piece of rock melon.

Rock melon is a wonderful cleanser and the quickest I know. If you like to eat garlic but don't like to share the aftertaste or the smell, eat some rock melon. A couple of slices and it will be completely gone. I love garlic, so I often eat half a rock melon the next morning to really clear away the smell and taste of the garlic or onion–but gone it will be, in a couple of minutes.

Real coffee; coffee beans are great blood cleansers as well. When you go out for coffee, have a Long Black instead. But don't add sugar.

Water Water Water. Keep in mind this—**feelings that indicate thirst and hunger are very similar**. So if you feel hungry, have a big glass of water before you snack on something. Then wait. Many times you will forget that you were hungry for an hour or more. This is because in actual fact, you were thirsty not hungry. The more dehydrated you are the more difficult it is to tell the difference.

If you are not sure if you are getting enough water, look at your wee. Your urine should be clear; a slight yellow tinge is OK. Remember also to check before you take vitamins, as the B group will darken your urine substantially. If your urine looks more the colour of apple juice or is slightly green, then you are in serious, even urgent, need of hydration. If you get a lot of headaches it could simply be due to a lack of hydration.

Don't drink water with your food. ONLY HALF AN HOUR BEFORE OR AFTER. Water dilutes your gastric juices which slow down how quickly the food is broken down in your stomach. Remember you need your food to move through the stomach and intestines and bowels as quickly as possible so as not to have time to go off.

**To increase your metabolism, eat regularly.
Not often—*<u>regularly</u>*.**

Eat at the same times every day so that your body can learn to trust that it will be fed on time and will not need to store any energy for later. This is especially important for people who tend to skip meals. If I find myself busy at work, I will at least stop for a quick meal replacement vitamin drink or a piece of fruit.

Don't ever skip breakfast. This first and most important meal of the day breaks your overnight fast and sets up your metabolic rate for the day.

If it suits you, eat often. That way you only need light meals. Rather than have two sandwiches for lunch, have one sandwich at 10:30 and the other at 2:30. This really works, especially if you had breakfast at 6:30 or earlier. You don't want to stretch your tummy, just fill it. Your body will begin to metabolize faster and faster as it will, in a few short days, realize that it doesn't have to store any of the energy you give it. It can utilize or eliminate everything, as it knows it is getting regular food. OH and you'll wake up hungry even starving some mornings.

Daily Routine Example

This routine is great for increasing metabolism
-
Wake up in the morning and immediately re-hydrate and drink a glass of water left on your bedside the night before and Streeeeeetch

Have a shot of liquid vitamins or take vitamin pill
Boil kettle and make ACV & Honey drink
Half-hour later have breakfast.
If you are on your way to work by now, you may need to have
a liquid breakfast that you can take with you.

- Half-hour later have a glass of water

- Two hours later have a glass of water

- Half-hour later have a morning snack

- Half-hour later have a glass of water

- Two hours later have a glass of water

- Half-hour later have lunch

- Half-hour later have a glass of water

- Two hours later have a glass of water

- Half-hour later have an afternoon snack

- Half-hour later have a glass of water

- Two hours later have a glass of water

- Half-hour later have dinner

Two hours after dinner have a glass of water, and go to bed
with another glass of water ready to drink in the morning. If
you are concerned about dust or bugs, put a lid or a coaster on
top of the glass.

So the rhythm to eat and drink water is:
½ hour before eating drink water
½ hour after eating drink water
2 hours later drink water
½ an hour later eat
½ an hour later drink water
2 hours later drink water
½ an hour later eat

Here it is again with times, but I wanted you to read it like that to get the rhythm. This is basically my routine.

6:30–07:00
wake up * drink water (1) * stretch * vitamins * ACV & H Drink
If you exercise, now do so and drink water halfway through. Once you get used to the routine you will be able to get up earlier, do the first above in about 15 minutes, and then that leaves you time to do an exercise DVD before breakfast.

07:30
Eat Breakfast

08:00
Glass of water (2)

10:00
Glass of water (3)

10:30
Light Lunch

11:00
Glass of water (4)

13:00
Glass of water (5)

13:30
Light Lunch

14:00
Glass of water (6)

16:00
Glass of water (7)

16:30
Snack

17:00
Glass of water (8)

If you exercise in the evening, do it now and have a glass of water halfway though. If not, just do the Pilates 100 before dinner.

19:00

Glass of water (9)

19:30
Dinner

20:30
Enjoy a cup of Green Tea to aide digestion

2 hours after finishing eating dinner
Glass of water (10) go to bed or relax

Note that you have had at least 10 glasses of water, plus more if you are exercising.

This diagram may help you see the rhythm:

	6:30	7:30	8:00	10:00	10:30	11:00	13:00	13:30	14:00	16:00	16:30	17:00	19:00	19:30	22:00
Water	▓		▓	▓		▓	▓		▓	▓		▓	▓		▓
Food		▓			▓			▓			▓			▓	

This shows that you are eating regularly every three hours with plenty of water in between.

Also, please note that my day rarely goes exactly to schedule. Plus, I haven't allowed time for getting organised for the day and going to work. I actually usually get up at 5:00–5:30 and am at work by 7:00. Usually by 10:30 in the morning I am starving and realise I haven't had my glass of water at 10:00, so

I have one and have to wait until 11:00 for my first lunch. Then I will have my next water half an hour later and the next one only one and a half hours later to get back in time.

Also, my afternoon snack is usually when I get home–whenever that is, but I try to leave a couple of hours until dinner. Or just have dinner really early. If I don't get home till after 6 PM I have dinner then.

Food Ideas For You To Enjoy For A Good Two-Week Cleanse.

Breakfast: Try to make breakfast as substantial as you can handle. This is when I love to have Oats–the ones with apple, honey and sultanas is yum, and I add low fat soya milk and I don't need extra sweetener. Natural (NOT TOASTED) muesli is also good. I also love avocado on a slice or two of toast with alfalfa sprouts and a hint of chilli on heavy wholemeal bread.

Lunch: If you do split your lunch in two then it is easy to make or buy two sandwiches and eat one at 10:30 and one at 13:30. Often I will have a sandwich for the first lunch and a soup for the second. Otherwise, for your first lunch or morning snack, have fruit, dried or fresh. If you can, put some fruit and yoghurt into a zooza to make a fruit smoothie/desert yummy thingy.

I like to get my carbohydrates out of the way early in the day and you should too, or at least by 2 PM. It is easy to stir a dip together cut up some veggies and enjoy, add herbs, Indian spices or chilli to get the flavour hit you are used to getting from salt. Do what it takes to make your food yummy for you.

Eat and enjoy your food, you should smile when you eat it is supposed to make you happy. If you enjoy what you prepare it is not hard work at all.

Afternoon or before dinner snack: If I am not cleansing I will have cheese and biscuits with a glass of wine but otherwise I will opt for stuffed olives and a mineral water but if I really need my cheese I will use sliced cucumber to replace the biscuits.

Dinner: Whilst cleansing, salad with something light such as tuna. Or soup. If you want, drop me a line and I can direct you to a fabulous soup recipe or salad ideas.

Please contact me if you are confused or need clarification on anything I have discussed here. There are no side effects to eating and drinking like this, but you will find that you do a 'number one' more often, as the water is flushing straight through you–especially the one you have when you haven't eaten for two hours; unbelievably refreshing for all your internal organs.

Your body will LOVE you!

And remember, sit down when you eat, eat slowly, and chew your food well.

You may be one of those many people who often complain that you just don't feel hungry in the morning, and don't get hungry all day, and can easily go without meals. THIS IS WRONG and should be addressed immediately.

If you are not hungry, especially in the morning after you probably haven't eaten for ten or so hours, then you definitely have a sluggish metabolism that needs a severe pep up. If you find it really difficult to eat breakfast, don't force yourself; start small. Start with 6 grapes and a juice if you must, start with one grape, <u>but start eating breakfast now!</u>

On the other hand, you may be someone that says, "I can't possibly have all that to eat so many times during the day. If I just eat one cracker or just look at food I put on weight". Well any wonder (!!!!) all you've given your body to function on is one nutrient poor cracker with little or no value, and so your body has no choice but to store it and hope for the best.

Now it is important to note that whilst on this eating pickup agenda, you will find that you will get hungrier and hungrier between meals, and this is a good sign and means that your metabolism is indeed picking up. Keep up the water intake and you won't suffer from feelings of hunger hardly at all.

But try not to snack in between or have larger meals. Just stick to your routine and remember that when you are hungry, you are losing weight. BUT NEVER EVER be hungry for more than an hour or two maximum. I have my own little rule that if I am trying to lose weight and I feel hungry, I have a big glass of water and wait for one hour.

I know it sounds boring, but eating sensibly really is clever. There is nothing wrong with sugar, fat or carbohydrates, they are all good and REQUIRED for your body's normal functioning. Remember, you want every cell to be balanced and working to its ultimate ability, then you WILL BE HEALTHY.

And remember to close your sphincter before you drink sugary, fizzy or alcoholic drinks.

Grazing all day is a common school of thought for increasing metabolism, but your body and its system really needs to do the whole 'hungry then satisfied' thing–**routine and rhythm are what your body loves.**

Please don't be fooled by foods that claim to be low in fat. They may well be, but don't buy them simply because this is stated on the label. Often the process that the food goes through to remove some of the fat leaves chemicals in the food which is worse that the fat content.

If in doubt, leave it out; natural is often better than low fat, low salt, or low carbs.

See what else is in the product; it may be much worse than fat. Of foods that claim to contain fruit, this may be true, but what else is in the product? It could vastly outweigh the benefits of the fruit, and be bad for you.

Here is some important information that may surprise you:

1 gram of protein	=	**4 calories**
1 gram of carbohydrate	=	**4 calories**
1 gram of alcohol	=	**7 calories**
1 gram of fat	=	**9 calories**

Hello! 9 calories for fat is the highest of all four. 9 calories is nothing you'd probably burn that taking a pee! The point is none of the four types of food are bad; it is the unnatural products that **your body does not recognise or need that cause all the trouble**.

There has been so much huff n puff over the last decade about high protein, low carb diets, and yet the **calorie count of protein and carbohydrates are EXACTLY the same!**

Just eat your carbs earlier in the day, as it takes a lot of energy to burn those. Carbohydrates are chains of sugar molecules, after all, and we need them.

Ask any athlete if they would consider have a diet lacking in carbs. They would look at you like you were mad.

BODY BRUSHING AND YOUR BLOOD

Borrowing the idea of Body Brushing from the Egyptians of thousands of years ago, I have always held this treatment in high esteem. This is such a valuable part of this treatment that I implore you to find yourself a body brush as soon as you are able. I have always found that the better brushes readily available at The Body Shop and from Bernard Jensen. If you have trouble obtaining one email me urgently and I will get one of mine to you.

Any natural fibre brush is satisfactory, but do try to get a cactus fibre one for stimulation and durability (they last for years and years). In fact I am so serious I want you to put this book down, grab your car keys, and go get one so you can start straight away.

Body brushing does many things that are of great benefit to your body's functions. It is extremely stimulating, and will bring that beautiful clean blood into those outer areas to bring oxygen and nutrients to assist in the cleansing of the cellulite.

Before I go in to the many benefits of body brushing, let me explain in very simple terms the blood and lymphatic system. It is very important for the blood to be as clean and free flowing as possible. This is why I insist on you drinking blood cleansing drinks such as the ACV & honey or the green tea or both as I do.

Basically the blood carries the good stuff digested from what you eat to where it is needed. The lymphatic system carries the bad stuff away to be eliminated. That is is insanely simplified but hey that is really all you need to know. Why complicate things?

Therefore both systems; the blood and the lymphatic, need to be operating at their optimum levels. It is almost a waste of time to have all your eliminatory organs all working beautifully if the lymphatic system is not bringing them the waste. Everything needs to be in sync.

Body brushing stimulates both these circulatory systems, and more specifically, the movement of the fluids. By increasing the circulation, the delivery of good stuff via the blood–essential nutrients and oxygen–is also increased. So even if you are eating well it is extremely important for those nutrients that are digested and metabolized to actually get to the organs and cells in your body that require them.

Similarly, the lymphatic system's fluids must also be stimulated to flow in order to carry waste such as toxins (cellulite) to the eliminatory organs where they can be exited from the body forever.

A quick way to verify you circulation is simply by looking at the colour of your lips. The pinker they are the better your circulation. If your lips are very pale without lipstick then you need to look at a possible circulation problem and vitamin intake. [Omega 3 will help support your heart and blood vessels. Antioxidants are also important here make sure your food intake includes berries and grapes (or have a glass of red!)].

When you first get your brush you will find it incredibly prickly and scratchy and will only just be able to make contact between brush and skin with the slightest of touches. So for your first brush, give it a soak. Just pop some warm water in the basin and pop the brush in bristles down. You only need enough water to cover the very ends of the bristles to soften them slightly. Overnight is the longest time, shortest being about one hour. I soaked my brush for a couple of hours about 20 years ago and I'm still using that same brush. So maybe every couple of hours let it dry and check it. You can always soak it some more but you can't harden the bristles up once they are soft. This brush will last you ages. You may find that you don't need to soak the brush at all, it just depends on your skin sensitivity. When I first brushed it was really painful so I soaked my brush. Last year I bought a new on and found I didn't need to soften the bristles.

So you want to brush until your skin begins to glow pink. Not very pink, more of a blush. DO NOT brush yourself red raw. Just brush enough to bring the blood to the skin. You will see your legs blush slightly; it is not super obvious. At first this will take some time, especially if you are prone to poor circulation. So do at least ten strokes in each spot and then check.

The blush may take a little time to show but you are aiming for an instant blush after ten brush strokes. You can then monitor your circulation, as it will increase and speed up as you brush, as your thighs will get pink faster. You will at first only get pink in a couple of odd spots. Where it doesn't come through this is where your cellulite is thickest. And it is difficult for the blood to penetrate.
Soon you will get that nice even blush that you want.

To brush, use long strokes. No need to press hard, and ALWAYS BRUSH IN THE DIRECTION OF THE HEART. Every stroke must be towards the heart, as this direction is what stimulates. The brush strokes need to be long and firm, just like brushing a horse.

(Little tip. If you want to massage someone to relax them, direct your strokes away from the heart–to stimulate go towards the heart.)

Start with the bottom of your feet, then the tops, then lower legs, then upper; pay particular attention to the bottom, then down across your shoulders away from your head, and up your arms beginning with palms and backs of your hands.

I don't generally brush my tummy. Its effect can be very strong. Very rarely, if I feel a bit sluggish after a pig-out at a steakhouse, I may very lightly brush three strokes moving across my tummy from the top bikini line up to the bottom of my ribs. But only very gently. This is good if you are trying to slim down.

If you are carrying extra weight around your middle do brush as it <u>will</u> help you so much. It is the sugar that gathers around your tummy as stored energy–again assisting the old beer gut or pot-belly. If all your stored energy is around your middle then you need to look at your sugar intake.

One more thing—brush in the morning. When I first started, I used to keep my brush on my bed side table on top of my alarm clock. I was so lazy and unmotivated I would reach for the brush and start to brush in bed. Starting with my feet, by the time I had done my lower legs and was up to my knees, I was awake and springing out of bed. The wake-up affect needs to be felt to be believed. If you are very sluggish in the morning and find it hard to get going, you will suffer no longer. Better than any coffee or stimulant on the market. Some of you will prefer to brush in the evening, but before a shower in the morning is most beneficial, plus I can't sleep after a brush or a coffee–you may be able to.

When you do the dry body brushing every morning, I need you to include the "*pit circles*" seven times. Leg, bikini and arm pits.

Do your lower legs first. Then do seven circles clockwise and then anti behind your knee where the lymph nodes are, you'll wake them up and unblock them.

Now brush your upper leg and buttocks and do the pit circles on your bikini line.
After you have done back stomach and then hands and arms; do the circles under your arms (armpits).

Stimulate all these nodes by doing the pit circles with the brush.

The lymphatic system carries waste to these nodes ready for the final stage of elimination. So these nodes must be clear and stimulated all the time. For those of you who have suffered great illness (perhaps pneumonia), the lymph nodes have been extremely stressed eliminating poisons. Now when you get a simple cold or allergy you feel your nodes flair up straight away. Sometimes you may feel the nodes on your neck swell up but you are not feeling sick. This means that your body is doing it's job very well and fighting and eliminating before you even feel sick symptoms, this happens all the time but if you are in tune and feel your nodes when they swell up help your body but cleansing to assist.

It is very important to do the pit circles with the brush, seven clockwise and then seven anti; first in each leg pit and then your bikini line, then the arm pits. This will stimulate your lymph nodes and activate them. When you first do this, well OK, when I first starting doing this, I reckon only about five bristles came into contact with my arm pits but I did the seven circles nevertheless, squeeling at the same time–but boy, what a rush. If you experience a bit of a head spin don't worry. The arm pit circles are very stimulating and close to your brain. (A great way to get the blood to the brain, I have known people to do this before an exam).

You (most people do) may find the brush at first to be too prickly and it will hurt. I have had the same brush for years and years. But when I first started there was no way I could cope with the harshness of the brush. But you will get used to it and the benefits are priceless so do try to persevere.

The last place you brush is across your shoulders brushing away from your head, this will brush away your stressy energy and is a great thing to do to start your day off right.

When the skin as an eliminatory organ is clean and clear and working, it too, will eliminate toxins and cellulite. Sloughing off the dead skin with your brush will greatly assist the cleansing of this large eliminatory organ.

It is also essential that your skin is clean and clear to not only eliminate, but to take in the essential oils that will go to work on your cellulite. (More on this in the next chapter).

Always remember that your skin is not just there to keep all your bits together inside.

Your skin is a very large and functioning eliminatory organ.

General benefits of Body Brushing:
Tightens the skin; helps digestion; helps to remove cellulite; stimulates circulation; increases cell renewal; cleans lymphatic system; removes dead skin layers; Strengthen immune system; improves exchange between cells and stimulates the glands.

Convinced yet?

Please see photos to help you know exactly how to brush your skin organ clean.

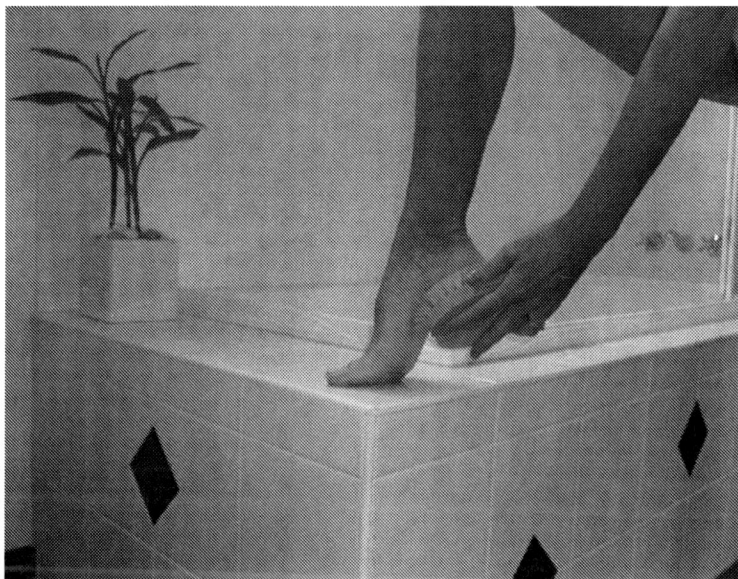

First brush up the bottom of your foot, then the top, and get in between your toes, too.

Then brush up your shins and calves in long steady strokes from your ankle to your knee, about ten in each spot and always towards your heart.
Then do the 'pit circles' behind you knees.

Next brush up your thighs from knee to bikini line, do the backs of your legs from the back of the knee to right up over your bottom.

Now do the pit circles on your bikini line. Remember 7 times anti then clockwise.

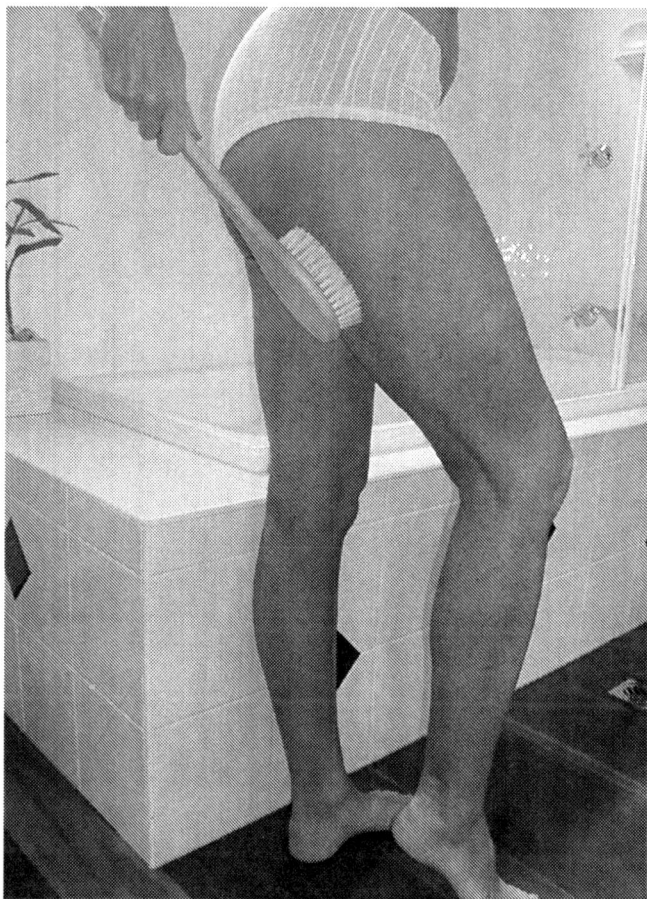

Brush long strokes from the knee to the hip.

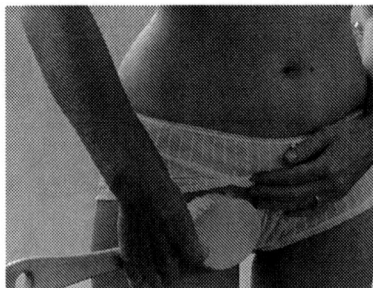

Once both feet and legs are done it is time to do your 'pit circles 7' clockwise then anti in your leg pit or bikini line.

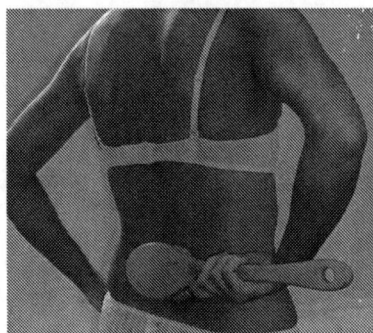

Now brush up the lower part of your back, and if you like, very lightly up your tummy, notice in the next photo I am only using the very tip of the brush.

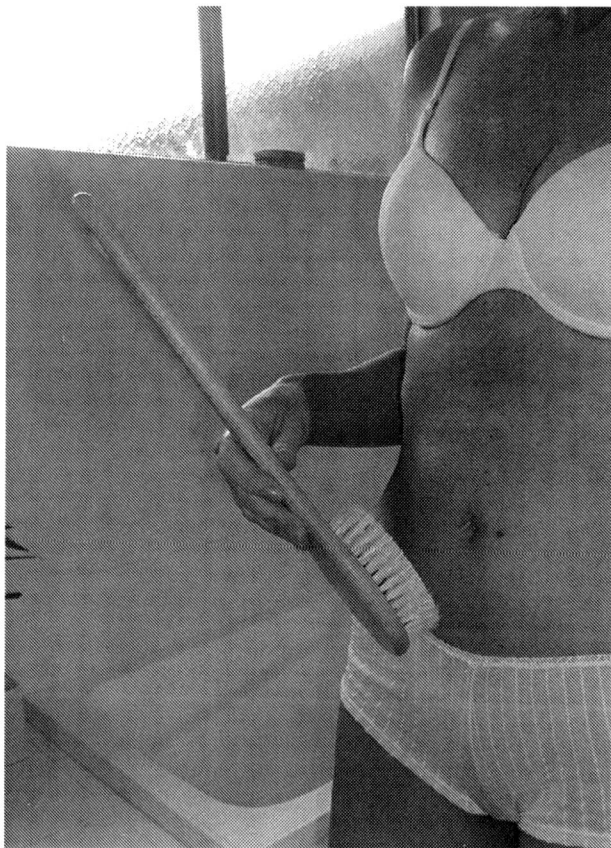

Now brush your hands—palms first—then the backs, then up your arms wrist to elbow, then elbow to shoulder in swift, long, steady strokes.

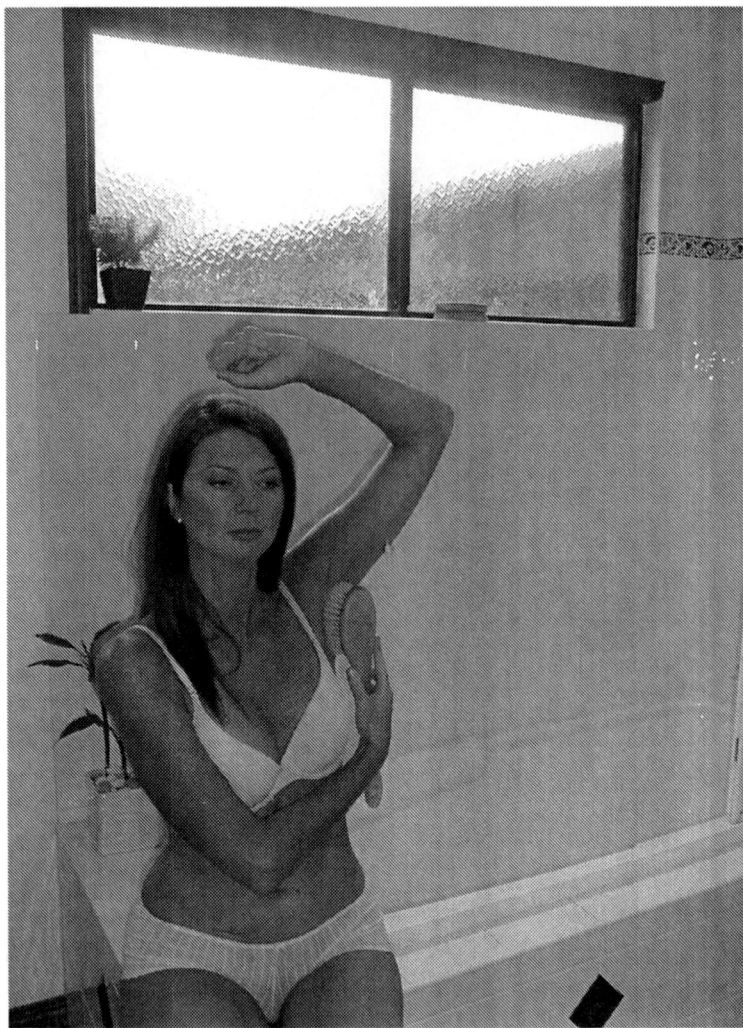

Do the 'pit circles', clockwise then anti, under your arms.

You will feel that (head) rush of circulation now if you haven't already.

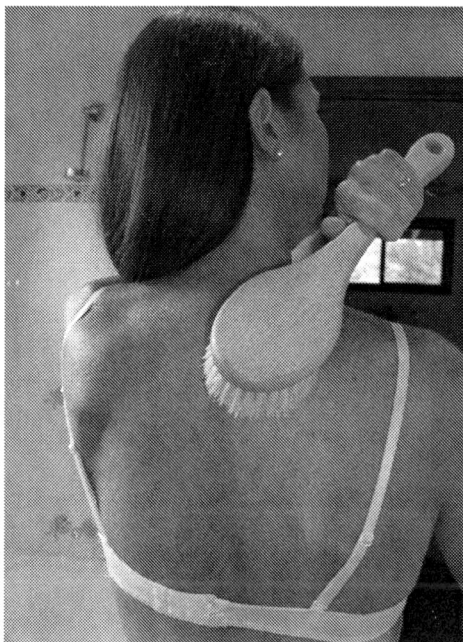

And lastly to finish off, brush across the top of your back from the spine out across the shoulders.

For specific cellulite areas, brush in that area for ten to twenty strokes or more until your leg blushes pink. This means you are encouraging and getting your blood into those cellulite areas to begin the cleansing process.

Remember to ensure you blood is clean of toxins by drinking apple cider vinegar, honey and hot water every morning.

OILS AND MASSAGE

Essential oils are a major part of your treatment. But it is also the easiest and the most enjoyable.

All you have to do with the oils is bathe in them a couple of times a week or as time permits. If you have a full house, tell them all that this book says you have to do it every night for the first month. That way you can escape for a little while every day.

Now for those of you who, like me, live in a small apartment, which unfortunately doesn't come with a bath, don't stop reading, as there are other ways to apply the oils, which I will get to shortly.

Firstly, though, I will explain to you the reasoning behind bathing in the oils, which will help the bathless of us understand what we will need to imitate.

The idea of bathing in the oils is simply to get the oils in through your skin. Your skin is an eliminatory organ and a rather large one at that. So it is really, really, very important that we have this eliminatory organ working at its absolute ultimate ability.

It takes about 15 to 20 minutes for the oils to seep through to start doing their work.

Yep, it is that simple, get the oils in and then let 'em go. Do not worry if you miss a week or two–the cellulite won't suddenly stop moving. This is good to remember in case you go through a period of time when you can't do all the aspects of the treatment, due to holiday, family or work commitments.

This is not a problem–just keep one or two of my directions on the go, for instance, take your psyllium husks on holiday with you and your body brush, this will keep things moving.

Now different oils do different things, but it is OK to mix them and they can all go in together. No need to do one at a time, but ok if you feel that you only need one of the oils in the bath. You may decide that your major weakness in your cellulite cleanse is circulation. So you may just want to have avocado oils with rosemary essential oil in your blend, this is fine for you to do, especially if you want to just target one area.

Most important to remember is that your essential oils must be administered to the skin only via carrier oil. **Do not apply essential oils directly on to your skin.** Only use without carrier oils in the bath or in a scent burner thingy.

Carrier oils do just that; carry the essential oils through your skin and into your body. And don't worry–mixing oils is the easiest thing in the world to do.

Carrier Oils I Recommend Are:

Olive Oil, and always cold pressed/from the first pressing. The first pressing contains a higher concentration of all the goodies found in olive oil. Often labelled 'extra virgin' olive oil, from the first pressing of the olives, which contains higher levels of antioxidants, particularly vitamin E and phenols, because it is less processed. Whether you use it in your food or your massage oils, olive oil is famous for aiding detoxification, which is what we need to help us rid our thighs of cellulite.

Grapeseed Oil is seriously beneficial for several reasons. Grapeseed oil has a neutral flavour and aroma, so is perfect to add to your massage oils and cooking, as it will not overpower as olive oil can.

Grapeseed oil is rich in vitamin E and antioxidants. The most powerful of these antioxidants is ProCyanidolic Oligomers, usually referred to as PCO's which are twenty times more powerful than vitamin C and fifty times more powerful than vitamin E!

The PCO in grapeseed extract is a bioflavonoid, which goes directly to the tissue, so it is easily absorbed. Grapeseed oil antioxidants are believed to prevent and control numerous ailments by safeguarding against the ravages of unstable oxygen molecules called free radicals. PCO's are thought to improve and help strengthen blood vessels, therefore improving blood circulation, which is what we are aiming for to help with the removal of our cellulite.

For the skin, grapeseed oil helps maintain elasticity and is used wildly in European skin treatments. You can get grapeseed extract in tablet and capsule forms, but please use it regularly to get the full benefit.

Sweet Almond Oil is also very popular and true to name. I believe it does just that—sweetens up your oil blend and for that reason alone it should be included. Sweet almond oil is also very nourishing and protects the outer layers of the skin. Use lesser amounts though as it does take a little longer than the others to sink in through.

I use mostly grapeseed and then add less of the others. See the massage oil recipe at the end of this chapter. Really, any oil is ok. Macadamia or any nut oil is good, but the benefits of the grapeseed and the olives are so good it is silly to leave them out of the equation. But, hey, experiment and mix up a different one every time. The aim is to find a mix that you enjoy and that suits your skin.

AVOCADO OIL!!!!! In caps and with exclamation marks as this is SOOOO important I really want you to take note. Avocado oil is the most wondrous carrier oil in the world as I know it, and is an absolute MUST to include in every oil you mix. You can easily test this by putting some olive oil and some avocado oil on your leg and see the avocado oil sink in quicker. By the way, 100% essential oils will sink into your skin eventually, no need to wash them off, and they don't stain either, although some of the darker oils may mark delicate fabrics and linen.

Also, very importantly, **never use mineral oils**. If you have mineral oil in your cupboard, throw it away NOW.

Always check any moisturizer, lotion or skin product to make sure it does not contain mineral oil. This is used extensively in cosmetics as it is a cheap bottle filler. Many companies appear to have the theory of that a little bit of essential oil, some vitamin C, some alpha-proxy-doohickies, fill 'er up with mineral oil and she'll be right, mate. WRONG!! Some products are simply 20% good stuff and the rest mineral oil or other fillers that will not penetrate the outer layers of the skin.

Mineral oil sits on top of your skin and seals it. This stops the skin from breathing; remember that death by paint scene in one of those James Bond flicks. They completely covered someone in gold paint who then died from suffocation–mineral oil acts the same way.

Your skin needs to breathe. Please don't suffocate your skin anymore.

OK, so now you have your carrier oil ready to go. Oils in dark brown bottles keep the best. Keep them somewhere dark and fairly cool, normally a bathroom cabinet will suffice. I live in the North of Australia and it is hot all year and mine have kept fine–mind you I have lost a few bottles of Merlot–*but that is a whole 'nother conversation.*

Now to select your essential oils. I will again recommend some oils for you, but if you found this book, no doubt you can surf the net or get to a book store and find others. There are hundreds of books out there on oils, so I really don't need to re-do what has already been done so well.

You can make up a bottle of oils to use that will last for a while or, you can get a little dip bowl and mix them up fresh every time, especially for massage, as it is easy to dip your fingers in to get more oil.

Here are my recommendations:

Juniper–which is famous for its cleansing properties (and that is what we are doing–cleansing, as opposed to dieting). This is such a good cleanser for your body it is oft referred to as a body purifier.

Most importantly for you, Juniper cleanses *and* is a diuretic, so provokes urine/waste excretion. At the same time, it is a stimulant, so is perfect for massage that is concentrated in certain areas. Whilst you rub the oils in or bathe in juniper, it will pass through your skin, cleansing the cellulite and encouraging its excretion along with other excess fluids.

Geranium–One purpose only and that is to budge fluid that your body is retaining. Plus it smells lovely. Geranium is, I believe very much, the under-appreciated oil. I always use this in cellulite blends, as it is extremely effective in loosening the hold on cellulite, making it available for elimination.

Rosemary–use this as much as possible as it is great for stimulating circulation and is essential for water retention. Most of us with cellulite have sluggish circulation, so try to include Rosemary in your blend.

Grapefruit—antiseptic, disinfecting, detoxifying, diuretic and skin toning this oil is beyond essential for any cellulite treatment.

At the end of the day you will mix a few before you get one that smells right. You are probably thinking, *Right, how on earth will I know when it smells right???* And this is difficult to explain so I will endeavour to do so by telling you a little ditty.

It does not matter who you are or what you are trying to achieve with essential oils–it must smell good to YOU. I can't stress this enough. We are all different and we all enjoy different smells, tastes, et cetera, which explains why there are sooo many scents on the market. If you smell any oil and don't like it's aroma—DO NOT USE IT!

It should *smell* good and make you *feel* good. Close your eyes and really let your sense of smell shine through. The connection between aromas and the brain are well documented and I encourage you to read up on this.

In the meantime, have you ever walked along a street and smelt a certain flower that reminds you of your Aunt's house when you were little? Or walked past a man who is wearing an aftershave that a previous partner used to wear–you haven't remembered the name of the aftershave but I bet you remembered the guy.

This is because the sense of smell is very closely linked to the brain and certain smells can bring a distant memory to life.

If you don't like the smell of an oil, you are possibly not meant to use it, and this may change as you do. And don't worry, lavender is one of THE most popular oils, and I admire it for its healing properties on burns, but I really don't enjoy its aroma and most people think I'm mad. My Mother loves it and I buy her lavender-scented things, but it is a bit too pretty and prissy for me and I can't wait to get them out of my car. So there is no need to feel something is wrong if you don't enjoy a popular scent.

Bathing in your oils.
The reason for bathing in oils is really quite simple. It is the easiest way to get the oils to where you want them enabling

you to target specific areas. The heat of the bath water opens up your pores of your skin and the pressure of the water helps to encourage the oils to move in through your opened pores.

When you are lying in the bath I want you to help the process with a little visionary assistance. You know that these oils will seep into your skin and go to work. So I want you to picture the oil surrounding the cellulite, and in doing so the cellulite simply loses its grip on the stored energy cell and slips away to be eliminated via your lymphatic system and then your eliminatory organs. The oil's properties encourage the cellulite to loose its stickiness, and make it easier for the body to flush away.

OK, so now for those of you who don't have a bath. I live in a very warm part of the world, so for me to get the oils in is very simple. I cover my target areas in oil and turn off the air conditioner. The idea is not to get too hot though, and in fact you don't even need to be especially hot for the oils to pass into your skin. You don't want to be sweating, as we want stuff to go in, not out at this point. So you can just wear some loose track pants, or just hang out naked for a while. The advantage of not bathing is that you can apply the oil only to those parts that show signs of cellulite, for those of you with severe or long term cellulite, remember to check your upper arms also. I suggest a hot shower and application of oils to damp skin. That way your pores are still open and the oils will pass into the skin with ease.

When buying essential oils, please make sure that you are buying ***essential oils*** and not fragrant oils. Fragrant oils have their place in the world but not in this treatment. ONLY ESSENTIAL OILS WILL DO THE WORK for you.

MASSAGE

The main reason for massaging is to stimulate the cellulite prone areas and also to bring the blood into the cellulite-affected areas and to manually give them lumps a bit of a budge.

Do get professional massages if finance and or location permit. Ask them to use your oils or ask if they have a cleansing one, and tell them you want a stimulating, deep tissue, or lymphatic drainage type massage. Many masseuses have a range of oils; if they have a cleansing oil, ask them what is in it.

There are three main techniques that we will use to help manually move the cellulite under the skin. First stroking, then knuckling, and we'll finish off with twiddling.

Stroking: using the palms of your hands apply the oils by stroking up your thighs in long strokes but as fast as you can (you will find that massaging really firms up your arms as does the brushing). This will warm up your thighs ready for the oils.

Knuckling: use the first knuckles (first back from the nail) and making your hands into a claw. Pull both hands one at a time up your thighs in swift upward strokes. To explain swift, count each hand stroke with a one-two; one-two as opposed to a one cat and dog; two cat and dog. Or one Mississippi; two Mississippi; what ever takes your fancy.

Don't use too much pressure; the normal pressure of pulling your knuckles up your thighs will be enough. If you bruise, please wait until your bruises heal–wait a week if necessary and next time go much, softer, as bruising will only antagonise the cellulite. Knuckling will encourage the blood to come to the surface of your skin aiding circulation.

Thumb Twiddling: have you ever seen your Grandfather sitting in a rocking chair twiddling his thumbs? Ok, so me neither, but you have perhaps seen it somewhere before and this is what I want you to do. Twiddle or roll your thumbs over each other in a forward rolling motion so that when you rest your knuckles on your thighs your thumbs do tiny little strokes in an upward motion up your thighs. [Don't worry too much there is a photo of this]. Do gentle thumb twiddling directly on any particularly large lumps or bumps. This will help loosen them up for elimination.

Whenever you have time, leave the oils on to slowly soak into your skin. Essential oils will eventually sink right in, but at first this may take a longer time. Once your skin is really clear from brushing it will take a much shorter time, 15 minutes or so.

And please, always remember to be firm but don't be too hard to cause bruising. Where ever there is damage on the body, the fat cells tend to move to the injury to help support. If you have cellulite it will bring the cellulite with it. I have seen many women over the years that have had liposuction, and then later the cellulite forms around the scaring, more concentrated than any other areas. If you are undergoing a cellulite treatment that is bruising you, please cease that treatment immediately. If you wish to chat to me about this further, please drop me a line at <u>askbron@gmail.com</u>.

A good routine is to brush, shower and then massage.

Basic Massage/Bath Oil Recipe
for a 200 ml bottle

CARRIER OILS

Grapeseed Oil	140 ml
Olive Oil	40 ml
Sweet Almond	10 ml
Avocado Oil	10 ml

For an even more basic model you could simply fill a bottle with grapeseed oil and then add a big splosh of avocado.

ESSENTIAL OILS

Geranium	10 drops
Juniper	10 drops
Grapefruit	10 drops
Rosemary	10 drops

You may only wish to add two or three essential oils at one time for each mix, just choose the best ones for you from the descriptions in the Oils and Massage chapter. Smell each of the oils whilst you are at the shop and decide which you enjoy the aroma of the most. This oil will be the one you need the most. Therefore add 10 drops of each of the oils to your blend but **add 20 drops of your favourite essential oil.**

If you have an Aromatherapist close by you may be able to get him or her to add antioxidant into the mix.

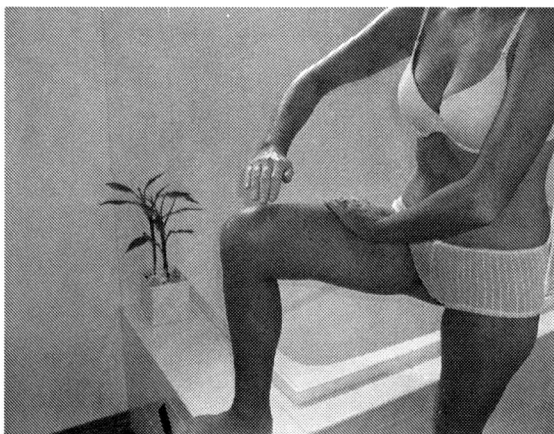

Step One: Stroking

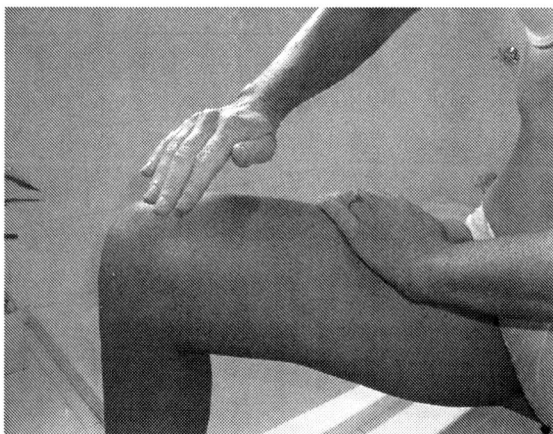

Stroking the top of the thigh

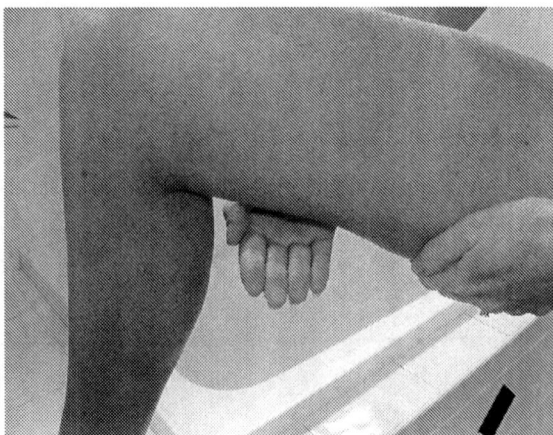

Stroking the back of the thigh

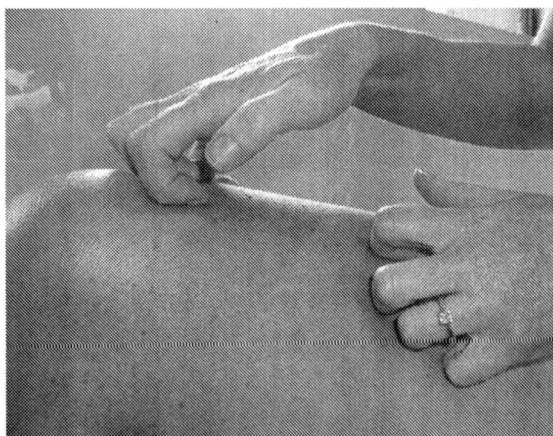

Step Two: Knuckling

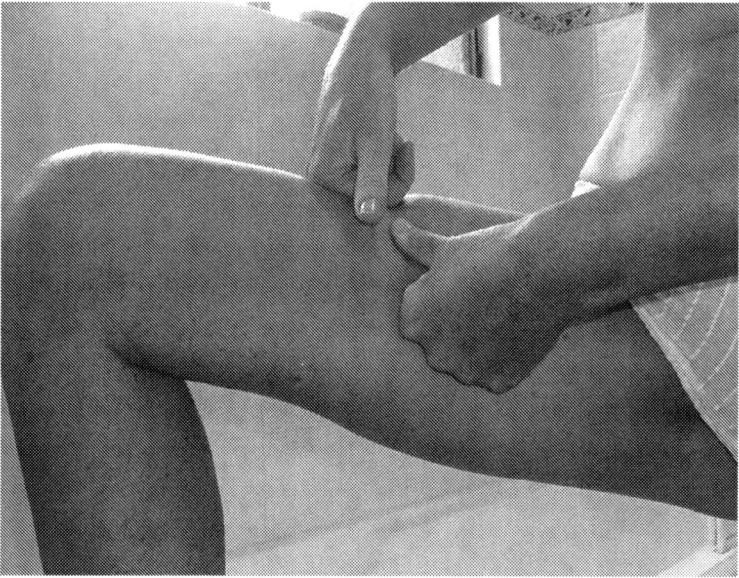

Step Three: Twiddling

AUTHORS NOTE

So now you know what to do. But where do you start?

I suggest you pick the most important things and start with them. Get yourself some psyllium husks and a body brush and start with that for a week or so. Drink the ACV + Honey drink to cleanse your blood.

If you are planning a holiday or you are very busy at work, do not put off starting at least some of the suggestions within this book. If you don't have time to do everything or you are away from home, just keep your brush with you and eat only natural, fresh foods where possible and drink water AND my favourite and most effective little tip—close your sphincter before you drink.

Also concentrate on making your and your family's life CHEMICAL FREE. Examine what you eat, what you wash your hair and body with; clean your house with and what cosmetics you put on to your skin organ. Start experimenting with natural alternatives to as many products as you can.

Please do contact me via email if you have any queries or you just want to share something with me.

I won't wish you good luck, as you don't need luck. It has nothing to do with it. It's completely natural and it works. Your body will love you for this change and will reward you for it.

So have a GREAT time. Get a friend involved with you for motivation if you want, or email me, but …
most of all relax, don't worry too much, and have some FUN

YOUR ESSENTIAL SHOPPING LIST

ACV & H Drink
Apple Cider Vinegar (aged in wood is smoother)
Honey

Lecithin
Capsule or grains. Capsules are more convenient as you can keep them
in your handbag for restaurant emergencies.
("yes I'will have the Peking Duck please")

Green or White Tea (bags OK)

Body Brush—Circulation and Tone
Made with Cactus Fibre–Hit the Body Shop Website

Bowel Cleanser—Digestion/Elimination
Psyllium Husks

Carrier Oils—to carry essential oils through skin to work on cellulite
Avocado

Sweet Almond
Grapeseed
Olive

Essential Oils—to work on your cellulite directly through your skin
Geranium to cleanse and drain wastes
Juniper to detoxify and dissolve fats
Rosemary for stimulation and water retention
Grapefruit for lymphatic system flushing

"You can achieve anything you want in life if you have

the courage to dream it,

the intelligence to make a realistic plan;

and the will to see that plan through to the end."

—Sidney A. Friedman

One final quote, which I heard just today. I have rushed to add to this edition. So if you are reading this page then I made it.

The quote below by Count Marichalar grabbed me, his words slapped my face and my eyes sprung open and a big smile spread across my face.
I now know more.

It is so simple. Make your choice.... .

"If you think you *might* give up;

You will

If you are absolutely certain,

that you will <u>never</u> give up;

You will not."

—Count Alvaro de Marichalar

COMMON QUESTIONS FROM READERS OF THE 2005 EDITION

Q: How much apple cider vinegar do I add to the hot water in the morning? My bottle says on or two teaspoons– is this right?

A: The easiest way is to fill a soup spoon with the vinegar tip it into the cup and then fill the same spoon with the honey, the remains of the vinegar will help it spread into the spoon better, then add hot water, from the tap is fine.

If you are drinking the premix (ACV and honey together) then two teaspoons is fine; but I do not recommend the premix as the taste is completely different to a fresh mix as it isn't just ACV & honey.

Q: Should I eat the psyllium husks in tablet form or spread over food in it's original form?

A: Eating the husks in their natural form should always be taken with two glasses of water–one with the psyllium stirred in and the other to wash the rest down. It is risky using the husks with food as you can not be certain of the amount of water available in the foods to ensure there is enough moisture for the husks to gel. It is OK to add the husks to foods for a little extra fibre i.e. add to your bread mix or cereal; but for the purpose of cleansing your intestines and bowel take the husks at night.

Many people add husks to their cereal, this is OK if you just add a little for extra fibre but not to replace taking the husks at night. If you take psyllium in the morning or during the day they can bloat your stomach, it is best to let them ease through your system while you sleep.

I personally being a bit lazy take the psyllium in capsule form and I keep them in the shower. Having a shower before bed is the last thing I do–I'm a bit funny about my sheets being clean–so I keep the container of capsules in the shower on the rack to remind me to take them before I go to bed.

Q: I heard that a raw food diet would be perfect to treat cellulite. I have a lot on my thighs.

A: Yes Eve the more natural state the food is in—the better.

Also don't buy precut veggies, as most of the vitamins have gone from them.

Soups are a great way to eat vegies in close to their natural state but any vitamins that have escaped are caught and held in the water.

Roasting vegies is also healthy, brush them with olive oil before you pop them into the oven.

Also remember to buy lots of different coloured vegetables to help you get a variety of vitamins

Q: I have had cellulite for as long as I can remember. I am a 42yr old mother of 2 teenagers. After purchasing your book, I have realised what I have been doing wrong all my life. White bread and potatoes were once upon a time, acceptable to eat. I lost quite a lot of weight years ago but the cellulite still remained. All I did was cut fat out of my diet and exercise and the weight fell off but the cellulite did not budge.

I am a fit person who eats well, or so I thought as when I cut fat out of my diet, I was thankful I could still eat my beloved bread and potatoes and are now paying the price.

After years of frustration, I signed up for the Endermologie treatments. $2500 and 26 session later, I have lost 7 cm off my bottom, my skin is smoother and the cellulite infected areas seem more loose and the dimpling has reduced somewhat but nowhere near what I expected.

Half way through my treatment, I had photos taken and I went home very depressed which led me to your book. I decided to research cellulite and after purchasing your book and following your advice, I have seen a big difference after just one month. My skin is much more supple and the dimpling has reduced.

Do you think I should continue with the Endermologie treatments? They are trying to get me to do 26 more sessions which I refuse. I was thinking of doing the maintenance program where you have the treatment every 2 weeks. What are your thoughts?

I have been body brushing, using essential oils, adding lecithin & psyllium husks to my diet and taking herbal pills along with eliminating white flour, potatoes and fizzy drinks. I tried the apple cider/honey drink and I just cannot stomach it but I will persist.

Awaiting your response.

Thanks

A: Those Endermologie treatments won't hurt you but are very expensive and won't achieve any better results than the brushing and the massage is. In my opinion Endermologie is possibly just trying to imitate the effects of massage and brushing. It would be much more beneficial to spend your dollars on having deep tissue or lymphatic drainage type of massages with essential oils. Much better value. See who is close to you and what type of massages they do that will be stimulating and therapeutic. And do that every two weeks or monthly. Very beneficial as it is the whole body that is treated not just one area. Ask them to use a cleansing oil or take your own if they don't for them to use on you.

I'm not sure about the dizzy spells, are you more tired than normal as well? This would be due to a lack of carbohydrates.

If you are so used to eating potatoes and white bread you still **need** some carbs in your diet. Good healthy carbs are available in:

- Whole grains
- Fruits
- Vegetables
- Legumes–beans, peas and lentils
- Dairy products

Q: I have been on your treatment for almost a month and I am already feeling better and can see changes in my thighs. My question is that I have a terrible flu and am wondering if it is connected?

Good question. You are very perceptive. It sounds like **you** are connected to your body. When you let your body cleanse and help it along, often and allergies that have been floating around your body finally come out and you experience the symptoms, commonly people get the flu when they cleanse as they never quite got rid of it when they had it. You could be experiencing some sort of allergy but I would consult a doctor if it persists for more than a week.

Are you taking vitamin supplements to assist your body to the change of diet? This is very important to ensure that you are getting what you need.

Q: I tried the psyllium for my constipation, I take it every morning and it does not help really and I feel bloated all the time.

A: Yes if you take it during the day it can make you feel bloated. If you are still bloated during the day after taking it the night before try adding more water as it may be gelling up too firm. Try to persist as it will clear but could take a couple of weeks if you need a good clearing. You may find that what you pass is pretty sticky and yucky—maybe don't look.

Q: Hi, I just have a question.
I am very constipated and I think that is why I have cellulite also.
I have been taking those fish oils, 2 capsules in the morning and 2 at night. It does not seem to work.
What do you recommend?

A: watch your water intake, is your urine clear. If not then you are slightly dehydrated and this can and will contribute to constipation.

Another thing that can encourage constipation are dairy foods. I love my cheeses so I make sure I have loads of fibre in my diet. And not just the grains and cereals but leafy green vegies have good fibre as well. Also stoned fruit is great to get things moving like nectarines or dates.

The other thing that is great for the bowels is walking (walk from your waist and hips not just your legs–this twisting action helps to get everything moving). Even just a quick walk will help loosen things up.
By the way the fish oil is wonderful—keep it up

Q: Thank you for your email. It was nice to hear from the person who wrote the material.

I have read through your notes and have just started with the Apple Cider and Honey cleansing in the morning, and after each shower, I am using Almond Oil/Avocado Oil/Geranium and Juniper oil mix on my thighs. I do try to dry brush beforehand, but my skin doesn't seem to go pink. Is this ok?

I am beginning to drink a little more of plain water–usually I have my weak coffee or tea with milk, no sugar so I really am forcing myself to try water. I am not a bubbles drinker.

I seem to fall into your second category person–circulation problem, so I will be working on improving the circulation by using some strategies you suggest.

Also could you please tell me if there are any side effects of using the Apple Cider–does it contribute to arthritis or anything?

A: OK so firstly no it is not OK that you skin doesn't go pink but is a definite sign that you have a circulation problem. How much are you brushing? To get my thighs pink (circulation is my thing too) I still have to brush hard like I'm brushing a horse, 10 strokes in each area to get my thighs to 'blush' pink. It may take a while before you get the blood to circulate to the skin in your thighs but keep persevering it is sooo worth it. It does take a while to get used to the brush too but if you brush, shower and oil on warm just showered and brushed skin you are going to really benefit from this routine.

If you are trying to drink water regularly for the first time it can be really hard, try squeezing lemon or lime juice into your drink but it is imperative that you provide water to your body on a regular basis. If you don't your body will store water but we are not camels, we have a regular supply of water so do it for your body even if you don't enjoy it at first.

I still have to keep a bottle on my desk and remind myself to drink it half an hour before I eat and then 2 hours later. I am always getting hungry and realising I haven't had my water so drink it and then wait half an hour. The water you drink two and a half hours after eating is the one that really flushes your system and is the most beneficial as there is no food to compete with and your body will love you for it. Make sure this one is straight with no juice.

As I also have circulation problems I could give you many tips on picking up your circulation but brushing first thing is a great way to wake the body up and some mornings I wonder if I would get going at all if I couldn't brush myself awake. Also try to do a little something to lift your heart rate before you eat. In the evening try to walk before dinner. At lunch time I'll try to do something, if at work I'll walk swiftly around the office or up and down a flight of stairs or at home I'll vacuum the house or something. If you are into exercise DVD's you must get Mari's Pilate's DVD's. Mari teaches you how to do the Pilate's 100 and I will often only do this before dinner it takes two minutes and is intense and it really helps increase circulation warming the body and burning calories and gets the heart rate up to help with metabolism.

The only side effect you may get from drinking apple cider vinegar is a rosy complexion. It is such a wonderful blood cleanser and imperative if you are brushing as you want clean blood to circulate around your body. And if anything it would assist arthritis but really potato juice is the best thing for arthritis as it's acid breaks down the crystals.

I hope this helps if you want any more information on the above or anything else please don't hesitate to email and keep up the good work.

So Marie: brush, shower and oil most days (four times a week is plenty). Eat real food. Lift your circulation before you eat to aid your metabolism and you will see results very soon within the first month. Remember once you cellulite starts to move it is difficult to stop it and it will look a bit worse for the second month but just when you think it's all going pear shaped you will see it really is going and has reduced substantially. Keep it up and you will keep your cellulite away for ever.

Q: I hope you had a lovely Christmas. I know its a very busy time of the year so I do apologise for sending small questions but you really are the best person to turn to. Just asking if my cellulite starts looking worse because its breaking down, how long is it usually before it starts looking better?
Since taking the psyllian Husks & lecithin (not sure of spelling) my
cellulite has gone a fair bit worse, especially on my arms & next to my
breasts. I feel hideous. I'm also looking at doing a course of detox spa
treatments which include an hour of massage, wrap & spa. **Do you think this might help?**

A: Yes your cellulite looking worse is a sign that it is breaking down and the firmer lumps remaining. I know it is an awful stage to go through but also one to celebrate. You cellulite is moving and once it starts it goes with great gusto. If you can get onto the essential oils now if you are not already doing so. Do some massaging and especially twiddling on those stubborn ones.

Going to a detox spa won't hurt but I would suggest deep tissue massage, or lymphatic drainage massage followed by a sauna most advantageous.

Keep up the good work. This awful stage should only last 2—4 weeks and then should start looking much better.

Please keep in touch.

Thanks for your Christmas cheer and I know you will have an amazing year next year. And don't ever apologise for little questions any time of day or night, which is why I am here just an email away. :-)

Q: I had the bath, and have been body-brushing and watching what I put into my mouth (this is the third day). I have also been taking the psyllium husks and boy, do they work! Just as you described.
I stood on the scales this morning and could barely believe I had broken the 73kg barrier–I was 72.8. I have been struggling with this for three months, bouncing around from 73 to 74.5kg but seemingly incapable of making those red digital numbers get any lower, even though I exercise. I am actually eating more food because I eat a good breakfast now. I hope this trend continues.
I have two more questions:
I bought lecithin GRANULES, not tablets ("German, GFO Free") and since there were no directions on the packet I wonder how much I should take? At the moment I

am having about 1 teaspoon of the granules with every meal. I don't know if this is not enough or too much.

Also I smoke cigarettes. When you suggest changing to raw tobacco, do you mean a brand like Drum?

A: Jill that is wonderful news, getting those results is motivation in itself—well done.

The granules of lecithin are fine and a teaspoon will be sufficient. The capsules are just more convenient that's all.

Yes unfortunately cigarettes are full of poisons and toxins that our body struggles to eliminate. Doing everything to assist your body's systems as you have started to do, will make the job of eliminating easier. Switching to a raw tobacco such as Drum will be a much healthier alternative, plus it gives you something to do with your hands if you smoke for your nerves and takes longer—you just can't grab a cigarette and light it you have to roll the thing and put the filter in first which means you will probably smoke less. There are also herbal cigarettes if you smoke for the 'drag' and relaxation, but they are more popular in America and I'm not sure where you would get them here, but your health food shop should be able to order them—give them a call.

You must be so pleased about your weight loss and breaking that barrier, this is because you have stopped your body fighting against you losing the weight as it is no longer in survival mode and getting fed regularly. Also cleansing away stored energy as opposed to dieting it away is the trick.

Q: What is the best time for me to massage the oils in–I don't have a bath?

A: Time for massaging depends on you and for how long you can massage. when I do a treatment (massage) on someone it takes 40 minutes to an hour—this depends on how clean the skin is from brushing and therefore how quickly the oils pass through the skin; and also how good your circulation is, i.e. how long it takes for your skin to blush pink from the massaging. It is easier to massage someone else than your self so when self massaging, to get the skin pink faster, brush firmly to bring the blood to the surface and then massage in the oils. It will take about 15—20 minutes for the oils to pass into your skin even in a hot bath so it may be beneficial for you to put the oils on and massage for as long as you can or as time dictates and if you are able to, leave the oils on to sink in at their own pace.

Q: Can you please explain to me when is a whole grain whole? What is a whole grain?

A: All grains start life as whole grains. In their natural state growing in the fields, whole grains are the entire seed of a plant. This seed (which industry calls a "kernel") is made up of three key parts: the bran, the germ, and the endosperm.

Q: I am a fellow 33 yr young aussie lady. I REALLY like your 'down to earth' E-Book on getting rid of cellulite!

It's GREAT to see a fellow Australian writing such helpful information I must say! I have tried SO many cellulite rubs etc not much good & very disappointing to say the least.

I only just bought your E-book online but have got the 'essentials' you suggest although I couldn't get the 'cactus' brush for the exfoliation I got the other type but looks just like the one you use in your book.

Anyway my question is if I am to have an essential oil bath (& yes I have all your suggested oils too) **How MANY drops of the oils do I use in the bath to make it effective? I gather I use just the essential oils not the carrier oil/massage oil mix in the bath?**

I have a spa bath so bigger than your average bath as well and I don't want the effects of the essential oils to be diluted if I don't use enough.

A: Thanks for your email and so sorry it has taken me so long to get back to you. Just found out that I'm pregnant and the shock at 41 is probably the same as if I was 16 so have been a little bit preoccupied at the moment. But I guess it goes to show that living fairly healthy means your body can do anything. Thanks also for the clapping smiley he is GREAT!

I hope your brush is OK. Does it make your skin go pink? It may take up to 20 brush strokes in one area to get your skin to blush when you first start. The brush bristles should be made from natural fibres i.e. cactus or from some poor beast and should be firm and a bit scratchy.

As you have all the oils you can add essential oils you can make a really potent mix by adding them directly to your bath.

You can also use a mixture of essential oils with your carrier oils as they are just so lovely for you skin. But to add directly I suggest about 6 drops of each essential oil and 10—12 of your favourite one in your spa bath.

If you brush, shower (with European micro cloth if you have one) you can keep your bath quite clean so that you can fill it up just a bit then have a soak then the next day top it up with hot water and you may be able to do this two or three times to save water and your essential oils.

Q: I'm only 20 years old and I have developed bad cellulite. does your treatment really work? what does it entail? thanks

A: Wow what a broad question … I will try to be brief in my response—I do tend to go on a bit, so will attempt to restrain. OK so the first thing I look at with a new client and the first thing **you** need to look at is WHY you are getting cellulite and why you are keeping it.

Even the BEST treatment in the world—even liposuction is useless unless you ascertain why you are getting cellulite.

You need to find your weakness—your cause. If you have say a lipo treatment and the cellulite and fat is literally sucked away, **it will still come back if you haven't fixed the cause.**

So once we know what your body's weakness is and what your personal cause of cellulite is then we can simply stop that cause.

Once you are not getting any more cellulite then we look at how to get your body to cleanse away the cellulite that you already have.

It all sounds simple and really, it is.

I have been teaching women how to get rid of their own cellulite for so long now—17 years or so and I am yet to meet someone I couldn't help. It is a little more difficult via the book but so far—2 years now—so good and I communicate with you like this and we do our best to talk via typed words.

As you are still young, can you remember when you first noticed your cellulite? If you can think back about 6 months before this time—did something dramatic happen in your life, maybe you lost a family member, maybe you left home = change of diet and environment.

If you can ascertain any of this it will help you work out why you have cellulite.

Have a think and get back to me. Usually people have had it for 10 or twenty years before they find me so we just look at the different things that may cause their cellulite.

There are many causes, you may have just one, you may have 4. The first step is to stop that cause.

Getting rid of the cellulite you already have is easy—just a simple cleanse and some clever tips and tricks to add to your life.

In the world of natural and 'alternative' medicine cleansing away cellulite is no biggy. Nearly all books on massage and essential oils list cellulite as something that is easily cured. They are not lying. Cellulite is easy to fix. Unfortunately the cellulite is a huge industry and is in fact now just that, it's own industry and many many people are making a lot of money and actually don't really want you to get rid of your cellulite as they would be out of business.

They know that even if a treatment works—you will be back as so will the cellulite. My live treatments cost about $1500 for the entire three months of three weekly treatments which is about as cheap as I can make it and the book I have kept the price down as well. It is my life's work to eventually rid the world of cellulite one lady at a time and to make it affordable for the wealthy and for those who are not.

Have a think about what I have emailed you and I hope to hear from you soon.

Thanks for reading

Read this book every two years or so

I still do

—Bronwyn

eBOOK INSTRUCTIONS

I hope these help a little–just in case you are not familiar with. pdf documents.

To view pages down the left side of your screen click on the 'Pages' tab top left of the top of the page.

You can increase or decrease the size of the page tabs by clicking on 'Options' above the page thumbnails and selecting 'reduce' or 'enlarge' the size of the page thumbnails.

To widen or make narrow the page thumbnail pre-view on the left of the document page you are viewing run your mouse over the border in between until you see a double arrow instead of your normal cursor (the arrows are heading in opposite directions) and you can then click and hold and move your mouse and the border to the left or right narrowing or widening the window.

You can print one page (i.e the Shopping List p.85) or a specific number of pages by clicking on Option then selecting print pages. Within the 'print range' section choose and click to mark a circle current page–the current page you are viewing–or type in from and to what pages you want (i.e The Top Ten pages 35—47).

To go to a certain page or chapter check the Contents (p.5) press the keys Shift and Ctrl together (with left hand)and the letter N (with right hand fingers–or do it all with your right hand if you're clever in that motor skills way;-). A little box will pop up in the middle of your screen. Type in the page you want and click on the OK button or hit your 'Enter' key if the 'OK' button is highlighted.

To get to the 'How to Pages' click the Shift key and F1 together. To close click on the 'Hide' tab at the top of the How To window.

To get to 'Adobe Reader Help' for a multitude of answers and assistance click on Help and the very top of your screen on the top toolbar and from the drop down menu select 'Adobe Reader Help'. On the left of this window you will see at the top the tabs Contents, Search and Help.

If you want to print of the entire document please feel welcome to do so or email me to find out where you can purchase the paperback version. As there are 100 pages you may want to choose the option of printing on both sides of the paper thus saving a small tree.

ABOUT THE AUTHOR

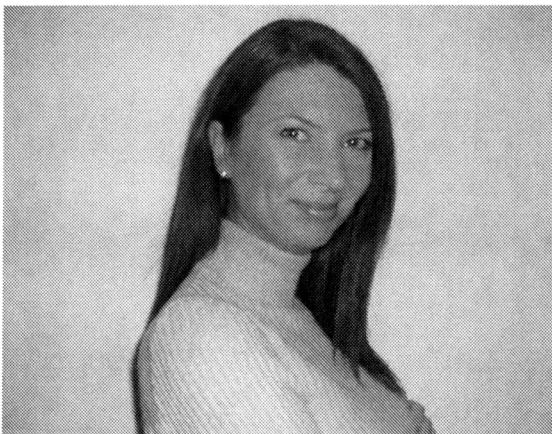

Bronwyn M. Hewitt is: certified in Massage and Health and Nutrition. Bronwyn had cellulite and set about investigating treatments, finding none that worked she decided to develop her own treatment which does. Combining several tried and tested natural therapies Bronwyn created *The Ultimate Cellulite Treatment* helping Australian women for 17 years.

978-0-595-46586-6
0-595-46586-2

Lightning Source UK Ltd.
Milton Keynes UK
28 April 2010
153469UK00001B/31/A

9 780595 465866